PROTEIN BASED DRUGS
A Techno-commercial Approach

PROTEIN BASED DRUGS
A Techno-commercial Approach

by
Dr. Chiranjib Chakraborty
Manager-Biotechnology (R&D), Glenmark Laboratories, Mumbai;
(Previously—Research Scientist, Biotechnology,
Macleods Pharmaceuticals Ltd., Mumbai;
Lecturer, Deaprtment of Industrial Fish and Fishery, Burdwan Raj College,
Burdwan, West Bengal, India)
&
Rajesh Jhingan
Vice-President- Glenmark Laboratories;
(Previously- International Business Head, Kee Biogenetics & Cimmco Birla Ltd.)

2005
BIOTECH BOOKS
Delhi - 110 035

ISBN 81-7622-107-4

Published by : **BIOTECH BOOKS**
1123/74, Tri Nagar,
Delhi - 110 035
Phone: 27382765
e-mail: biotechbooks@yahoo.co.in

Showroom : 4762-63/23, Ansari Road, Darya Ganj,
New Delhi - 110 002
Phone: 23245578, 23244987

Laser Typesetting : **Classic Computer Services**
Delhi - 110 035

Printed at : **Chawla Offset Printers**
Delhi - 110 052

PRINTED IN INDIA

Preface

When we started this book, our plans were to help those not yet captive of the field of protein based drugs on technical aspects only. Some thoughts came to our mind to include also global view and commercialization potential vis a vis Pharma-Biotech industry as on today. This should be a pleasant and enlightening surprise for readers who have wondered what all the fuss is about.

Today the world market for therapeutic proteins is over USD 22 Billion and India represent just 1 percent , however India is poised for exponential growth in next five years and expected to take global market share of 10 percent.

In our several sections of the book we have addressed not only about the technical aspects pertaining importance of proteins, protein based drugs and their production process, synthetic peptides, quality control and characterization, delivery systems and formulation development but also on present world scenario, regulatory aspects, therapeutic innovation and intellectual property rights and guide to new entrepreneurs.

Our goal in this effort and also perhaps matter of great concern. Technical expertise is not sufficient or at times may be of insignificant importance unless or until one is commercially as strong. Techno-Commercial is the key word today and the cross-fertilization of these two is must.

We gratefully acknowledge the sources of many ideas in the text that we have adopted in the book.

We wish to express our thanks to Mr. Anil Mittal, Director, Daya Publishing house for providing us the excellent opportunity. Criticisms and suggestions are always welcome from the readers for further improvement of our book.

Last and not the least we wish our thoughts and efforts put together shall surely benefit the readers.

Dr. Chiranjib Chakraborty
Rajesh Jhingan

Contents

Chapter 1

Biotechnology and Proteins

One of the major challenges for people who wish to know and work in the domain of molecular biology is becoming conversant with the daunting intricacies of existing biological knowledge and its extensive technical vocabulary. Questions about the origin, function, and structure of living systems have been pursued by nearly all cultures throughout history, and the work of the last two generations has been particularly fruitful. The knowledge of living systems resulting from this research is far too detailed and complex for any one human to comprehend. An entire scientific career can be based in the study of a single biomolecule. Nevertheless, in the following pages, we attempt to provide enough background for people to understand much of the biology discussed in this chapter. This chapter provides the briefest of overviews; We can only begin to convey the depth, variety, complexity and stunning beauty of the universe of living things.

Much of what follows is not about *molecular biology* per se. In order to explain what the molecules are doing, it is often necessary to use concepts involving, for example, cells, embryological development, or evolution. Biology is frustratingly holistic. Events at one level can effect and be affected by events at very different levels of scale or time. Digesting a survey of the basic background material is a prerequisite for understanding the significance of the molecular biology that is described in the book. In life, as in cognition, context is very important (1).

About Life

No simple definition of what it is to be a living thing captures our intuitions about what is alive and what is not. The central feature of life is its ability to reproduce itself. Reproductive ability alone is not enough; computer programs can create endless copies of themselves-that does not make them alive. Crystals influence the matter around them to create structures similar to themselves but they're not alive, either. Most living things take in materials from their environment and capture forms of energy they can use to transform those materials into components of themselves or their offspring. Viruses, however, do not do that; they are nearly pure genetic material, wrapped in a protective coating. The cell that a virus infects does all the synthetic work involved in creating new viruses. Are viruses a form of life? Many people would say so.

Another approach to defining "life" is to recognize its fundamental interrelatedness. Organisms came to differ from each other, and to reach modern levels of complexity through *evolution.* Evolution has three components: inheritance, the passing of characteristics from parents to offspring. Evolution is the key not only to defining what counts as life but also to understanding how living systems function.

Evolution is a cumulative process. *Inheritance* is the determinant of almost all of the structure and function of organisms; the amount of variation from one generation to the next is quite small. Inheritance alone, however, is not sufficient for evolution to occur; perfect inheritance would lead to populations of entirely identical organisms, all exactly like the first one.

Although our understanding of the molecular level of life is less detailed, it appears that this diversity is echoed there. For example, proteins with very similar shapes and identical functions can have radically different chemical compositions. And organisms that look quite similar to each other may have very different genetic blueprints. All of the genetic material in an organism is called its *genome.* Genetic material is discrete and hence has a particular size, although the size of the genome is not directly related to the complexity of the organism. The size of genomes varies from about 5,000 elements in a very simple organism to more than 10^{11} elements some higher plants; people have about $3x10^9$ elements in their genome. Despite this incredible diversity, nearly all of the same basic mechanisms are present in all organisms. All living things are made of cells (2).

Non-biologists often fail to appreciate the tremendous number of different kinds of organisms in the world. Although no one really knows, estimates of the number of currently extant species range from 5 million to 50 million. There are at least 300,000 different kinds of beetles alone, and probably 50,000 species of tropical trees. Familiar kinds of plants and animals make up a relatively small proportion of the kinds of living things, perhaps only 20%. Vertebrates (animals with backbones: fish, reptiles, amphibians, birds, mammals) make up only about 3% of the species in the world.

Since Aristotle, scholars have tried to group these myriad species into meaningful classes. This pursuit remains active, and the classifications are, to some degree, still controversial. Traditionally, these classifications have been based on the *morphology* of organisms. Literally, morphology means shape, but it is generally taken to include internal structure as well. Morphology is only part of phenotype, however; other parts include physiology, or the functioning of living structures, and development. Structure, development and function all influence each other, so the dividing lines are not entirely clear. In recent years, these traditional taxonomies have been shaken by information gained from analyzing genes directly, as well as by the discovery of an entirely new class of organisms that live in hot, sulphurous environments the deep sea.

There are three most basic divisions: the Archaea, the Bacteria and the Eucarya. Eucarya (also called eucaryotes) are the creatures we are most familiar with. They have cells that contain nuclei, a specialized area in the cell that holds the genetic material. Eucaryotic cells also have other specialized cellular areas, called organelles. An example of organelles are mitochondria and chloroplasts. Mitochondria are where respiration takes place, the process by which cells use oxygen to improve their efficiency at turning food into useful energy (24).

Chloroplasts are organelles found in plants that capture energy from sunlight. All multicellular organisms, (*e.g.* people, mosquitos and maple trees) are Eucarya, as are many single celled organisms, such as yeasts and paramecia. Even within Eucarya, there are more kinds of creatures than many non-biologists expect. Within the domain of the eucaryotes, there are generally held be at least four kingdoms: animals, green plants, fungi and protists. From a genetic viewpoint, the protists, usually defined as single celled organisms other than fungi, appear to be a series of kingdoms, including at least the ciliates (cells with many external hairs, or cillia), the flagellates (cells with a single, long external fiber) and the microsporidia.

Now there is always a question arises in our mind that where do these variations come from? Before the advent of sex, variations arose solely through individual, random changes in genetic material. A mutation might arise, changing one element in the genome, or a longer piece of a genome might be duplicated or moved. If the changed organism had an advantage, the change would propagate itself through the population. Most mutations are neutral or deleterious, and evolutionary change by mutation is a very slow, random search of a vast space. The ability of two successful organisms to combine bits of their genomes into an offspring produced variants with a much higher probability of success. Those moves in the search space are more likely to produce an advantageous variation than random ones. Although you wouldn't necessarily recognize its sex when looking under a microscope, even some Bacteria exchange genetic material. How and when sexual recombination first evolved is not clear, but it is quite ancient. Some have argued that sexual reproduction was a necessary precursor to the development of multicellular organisms with specialized cells (3). The advent of sex dramatically changed the course of evolution. Whether or not it occurred as a result of the advent of sexual recombination, the origin of multicellular organisms led to a tremendous explosion in the kinds of organisms and in their complexity. This event occurred only about a billion years ago, about three quarters of the way through the history of life.

Proteins are the molecules that accomplish most of the functions of living cell. The number of different structures and functions that proteins take on in a single organism is staggering. They make possible all of chemical reactions in the cell by acting as *enzymes* that promote specific chemical reactions, which would otherwise occur only so slowly as to otherwise negligible. The action of promoting chemical reactions is called *catalysis*, and enzymes are sometimes refered to as *catalysts*, which is a more general term. Proteins also provide structural support, and are the keys how the immune system distinguishes self from invaders. They provide mechanism for acquiring and transforming energy, as well as translating into physical work in the muscles. They underlie sensors and the transmission of information as well.

All proteins are constructed from linear sequences of smaller molecules called amino acids. There are twenty naturally occurring amino acids. Long proteins may contain as many as 4500 amino acids, so the space of possible proteins is very large: 204500 or 105850. Proteins also fold up to form particular three dimensional shapes, which give them their specific chemical functionality.

Although it is easily demonstrable that the linear amino acid sequence completely specifies the three dimensional structure of most proteins, the details of that mapping is one of the most important open questions of biology. In addition a protein's three dimensional structure is not fixed; many proteins move and flex in constrained ways, and that can have a significant role in their biochemical function. Also, some proteins bind to other groups of atoms that are required for them to function. These other structures called *prosthetic groups.* An example of a prosthetic group is *heme,* which binds oxygen in the protein hemoglobin. We will discuss proteins in more detail again below.

Genetic material codes for all the other constituents of the the cell. information is generally stored in long strands of DNA. In Bacteria, the DNA generally circular. In Eucaryotes, it is linear. During cell division Eucaryotic DNA is grouped into X shaped structures called chromosomes. Some viruses (like the AIDS virus) store their genetic material in RNA. This genetic material contains the blueprint for all the proteins.

Knowledge of cells and tissues makes possible the functional accounts of physiology. For example, knowing that the cells in the bicep and in the heart are both kinds of muscle helps explain how the blood circulates. However, at this level of description, the work that individual cells are able to do remains mysterious. The revolution in biology over the last three decades resulted from the understanding cells in terms of their chemistry. These insights began with descriptions of the molecules involved in living processes, and now increasingly provides an understanding of the molecular structures and functions that are the fundamental objects and actions of living material. More and more of the functions of life (*e.g.* cell division, immune reaction, neural transmission) are coming to be understood as the interactions of complicated, self-regulating networks of chemical reactions. The substances that carry out and regulate these activities are generally referred to as biomolecules. Biomolecules include proteins, carbohydrates, lipids-all called *macromolecules* because they are relatively large-and a variety of small molecules. The genetic material of the cell specifies how to create proteins, as well as when and how much to create. These proteins, in turn, control the flow of energy and materials through the cell, including the creation and transformation of carbohydrates, lipids and other molecules, ultimately accomplishing all of the functions that the cell carries out. The genetic material itself is also now known to be a particular macromolecule: DNA.

In even the simplest cell, there are more than a thousand kinds of biomolecules interacting with each other; in human beings there are likely to be more than 100,000 different kinds of proteins specified in the genome (it is unlikely that all of them are present in any particular cell). Both the amount of each molecule and its concentration in various compartments of the cell determines what influence it will have. These concentrations vary over time, on scales of seconds to decades. Interactions among biomolecules are highly non-linear, as are the interactions between biomolecules and other molecules from outside the cell. All of these interactions take place in parallel among large numbers of instances of each particular type. Despite this daunting complexity, insights into the structure and function of these molecules, and into their interactions are emerging very rapidly.

One of the reasons for that progress is the conception of life as a kind of information processing. The processes that transform matter and energy in living systems do so under the direction of a set of symbolically encoded instructions.

The Molecular Building Blocks of Life

Living systems process matter, energy and information. The basic principle of life, reproduction, is the transformation of materials found in the environment of an organism into another organism. Raw materials from the local environment are broken down, and then reassembled following the instructions in the genome. The offspring will contain instructions similar to the parent.

The matter, energy and information processing abilities of living systems are very general; one of the hallmarks of life is its adaptability to changing circumstances. Some aspects of living systems have, however, stayed the same over the years. Despite nearly 4 billion years of evolution, the basic molecular objects for carrying matter, energy and information have changed very little.

The basic units of matter are proteins, which subserve all of the structural and many of the functional roles in the cell; the basic unit of energy is a phosphate bond in the molecule adenosine triphosphate (ATP); and the units of information are four nucleotides, which are assembled together into DNA and RNA.

The chemical composition of living things is fairly constant across the entire range of life forms. About 70% of any cell is water. About 4% are small molecules like sugars and inorganic *ions*. One of these small molecules is ATP, the energy carrier. Proteins make up between 15% and 20% of the cell; DNA and RNA range from 2% to 7% of the weight. The cell membranes, lipids and other, similar molecules make up the remaining 4% to 7% (2).

Energy

Living things obey all the laws of chemistry and physics, including the second law of thermodynamics, which states that the amount of entropy (disorder) in the universe is always increasing. The consumption of energy is the only way to create order in the face of entropy. Life doesn't violate the second law; living things capture energy in a variety of forms, use it to create internal order, and then transfer energy back to the environment as heat. An increase in organization within a cell is coupled with a greater increase in disorder outside the cell. Living things must capture energy, either from sunlight through photosynthesis or from nutrients by respiration. The variety of chemicals that can be oxidized by various species to obtain energy through respiration is immense, ranging from simple sugars to complex oils and even sulfur compounds from deep sea vents (in the case of Archaea).

In many cases, the energy is first available to the cell as an electrochemical gradient across the cell membrane. The cell can tap into electrochemical gradient by coupling the energy that results from moving electrons across the membrane to other processes. There are many constraints on the flow of energy through a living system.

Most of the chemical reactions that organisms need to survive require an input of a minimum amount of energy to take place at a reasonable rates; efficient use of energy dictates that this must be delivered in a quanta exceeding the minimum requirement only slightly. The energy provided for biochemical reactions has to be useable by many different processes. It must be possible to provide energy where it is needed, and to store it until it is consumed. The uses of energy throughout living systems are very diverse. It is needed to synthesize and transport biomolecules, to create mechanical action through the muscle proteins action and myosin, and to create and maintain electrical gradients, such as the ones that neurons use to communicate and compute. Storing and transporting energy in complex biochemical systems runs the risk of disrupting chemical bonds other than the target ones, so the unit of energy has to be small enough not to do harm, but large enough to be useful. The most common carrier of energy for storage and transport is the outermost phosphate bond in the molecule *adenosine triphosphate,* or *ATP*. This molecule plays a central role in every living system: it is the carrier of energy. Energy is taken out of ATP by the process of *hydrolysis*, which removes the outermost phosphate group, producing the molecule adenosine diphosphate (ADP). This process generates about 12 kcal per mole of ATP, a quantity appropriate for performing many cellular tasks. The energy "charge" of a cell is expressed in the ratio of ATP/ADP and the electrochemical difference between the inside and the outside of the cell (which is called the *transmembrane potential*). If ATP is depleted, the movement of ions caused by the transmembrane potential will result in the synthesis of additional ATP. If the transmembrane potential has been reduced (for example, after a neuron fires), ATP will be consumed to pump ions back across the gradient and restore the potential (6).

ATP is involved in most cellular processes, so it is sometimes called a *currency* metabolite. ATP can also be converted to other high energy phosphate compounds such as *creatine phosphate,* or other nucleotide triphosphates.

In turn, these molecules provide the higher levels of energy necessary to transcribe genes and replicate chromosomes. Energy can also be stored in different chemical forms. Carbohydrates like glycogen provide a moderate density, moderately accessible form of energy storage. Fats have very high energy storage density, but the energy stored in them takes longer to retrieve.

Proteins

Proteins are the primary components of living things, and they play many roles. Proteins provide structural support and the infrastructure that holds a creature together; they are enzymes that make the chemical reactions necessary for life possible; they are the switches that control whether genes are turned on or off; they are the sensors that see and taste and smell, and the effectors that make muscles move; they are the detectors that distinguish self from nonself and create an immune response. Finding the proteins that make up a creature and understanding their function is the foundation of explanation in molecular biology.

Despite their radical differences in function, all proteins are made of the same basic constituents: the amino acids. Each amino acid shares a basic structure, consisting of a central carbon atom (C), an *amino* group (NH_3) at one end, a *carboxyl* group (COOH) at the other, and a variable sidechain (R), as shown in Figure. For example, under biological conditions the amino end of the molecule is positively charged, and the carboxyl end is negatively charged. Chains of amino acids are assembled by a reaction that occurs between the nitrogen atom at the amino end of one amino acid and the carbon atom at the carboxyl end of another, bonding the two amino acids and releasing a molecule of water. The linkage is called a *peptide bond*, and long chains of amino acids can be strung together into polymers, called *polypeptides*, in this manner. All proteins are polypeptides, although the term polypeptide generally refers to chains that are shorter than whole proteins (7).

When a peptide bond is formed, the amino acid is changed (losing two hydrogen atoms and an oxygen atom), so the portion of the original molecule integrated into the polypeptide is often called a *residue*. The sequence of amino acid residues that make up a protein is called the protein's *primary structure*. The primary structure is directly coded for in the genetic material: The individual elements of a DNA molecule form triples which unambiguously specify an amino acid. A genetic sequence maps directly into a sequence of amino acids. It is interesting to note that only a small proportion of the very many possible polypeptide chains are naturally occurring proteins. Many proteins contain more than 100 amino acids (some have more than 4000). The number of possible polypeptide chains of length 100 is 20^{100} or more than 10^{130}. Even if we take the high

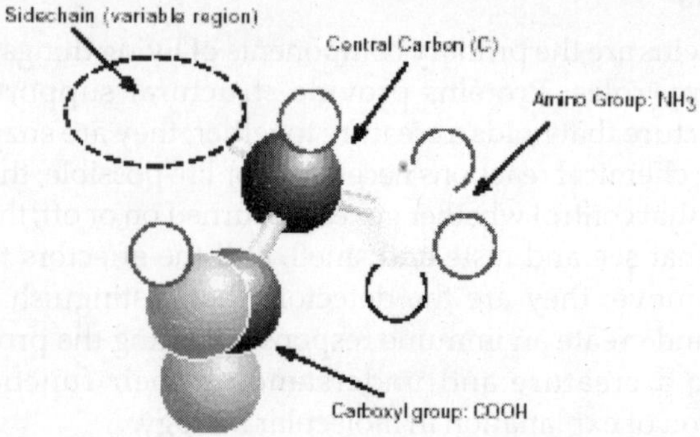

Figure 1.1: The Basic Chemical Structure of an Amino Acid.

estimates of the number of species ($5x10^7$) and assume that they all have as many different proteins as there are in the most complex organism ($<10^7$) and that no two organisms share a single protein, the ratio of actual proteins to possible polypeptides is much less than $1:10^{100}$-a very small proportion, indeed. The twenty naturally occurring amino acids all have the common elements. The varying parts are called *sidechains;* the two carbons and the nitrogen in the core are sometimes called the *backbone*. Peptide bonds link together the backbones of a sequence of amino acids. That link can be characterized as having two degrees of rotational freedom, the phi and psi angles. The conformation of a protein backbone (*i.e.* its shape when folded) can be adequately described as a series of angles, although it is also possible to represent the shape using the Cartesian coordinates of the central backbone atom (the alpha carbon). The dimensions along which amino acids vary are quite important for a number of reasons. One of the major unsolved problems in molecular biology is to be able to predict the structure and function of a protein from its amino acid sequence. It was demonstrated more than two decades ago that the amino acid sequence of a protein determines ultimate conformation and, therefore, its biological activity and function. Exactly how the properties of the amino acids in the primary structure of a protein interact to determine the protein's ultimate conformation remains unknown. The chemical properties of the individual, amino acids, however, are known with great precision. These properties form the basis for many representations of amino acids. Here is a brief summary of some of them. *Glycine* is the simplest amino acid; its sidechain is a single hydrogen atom. It is nonpolar, and does not ionize easily. The *polarity* of a molecule refers to the degree that its electrons are distributed asymmetrically. A nonpolar molecule has a relatively even distribution of charge. *Ionization* is the process that causes a molecule to gain or lose an electron, and hence become charged overall. The distribution of charge has a strong effect on the behavior of a molecule (*e.g.* like charges repel). Another important characteristic of glycine is that as a result of having no heavy (*i.e.* non-hydrogen) atoms in its sidechain, it is very flexible. That flexibility can give rise to unusual kinks the folded protein. *Alanine* is also small and simple; its sidechain is just a *methyl* group (consisting of a carbon and three hydrogen atoms). Alanine is one of the most commonly appearing amino acids. Glycine and alanine's sidechains are *aliphatic*, which means that they are straight chains (no loops) containing only carbon and hydrogen atoms. There are three other aliphatic amino acids: *valine, leucine* and *isoleucine.* The longer aliphatic sidechains are hydrophobic. Hydrophobicity is one of the key factors that determines how the chain of amino acids will fold up into an active protein. Hydrophobic residues tend to come together to form compact core that exclude water. Because the environment inside cells is *aqueous* (primarily water), these hydrophobic residues will tend to be on the inside of a protein, rather than on its surface. In contrast to alanine and glycine, the sidechains of amino acids *phenylalanine, tyrosine* and *tryptophan* are quite large. Size matters in protein folding because atoms resist being too close to one another, so it is hard to pack many large sidechains closely. These sidechains are also *aromatic*, meaning that they form closed rings of carbon atoms with alternating double bonds like the simple molecule benzene). These rings are large and inflexible. Phenylalanine and tryptophan are also hydrophobic. Tyrosine has a *hydroxyl* group (an OH at the end of the ring), and is therefore more reactive than the other sidechains mentioned so far, and less hydrophobic. These large amino acids appear less often than would be expected ifproteins were composed randomly. *Serine* and *threonine* also contain hydroxyl groups, but do not have rings. Another feature of importance in amino acids is whether they ionize to form charged groups. Residues that ionize are characterized by their *pK*, which indicates at what *pH* (level of acidity) half of the molecules of that amino acid will have ionized. *Arginine* and *lysine* have high pK's (that is, they ionize in basic environments) and *histidine*, *gluatmic acid* and *aspartic acid* have low pK's (they ionize in acidic ones). Since like charges repel and opposites attract, charge is an important feature in predicting protein conformation. Most of the charged residues in a protein will be found at its surface, although some will form bonds with each other (on the inside of the molecule called *salt-bridges*) which can provide strong constraints on the ultimate folded form. *Cysteine* and *methionine* have hydrophobic sidechains that contain a sulphur atom, and each plays an important role in protein structure. The sulphurs make the amino acids' sidechains very reactive. Cysteines can form *disulphide* bonds with each other; disulphide bonds often hold distant parts of a polypeptide chain near each other, constraining the folded conformation like salt bridges. For that reason, cysteines have a special role in determining the three dimensional structure of proteins. Methionine is also important because all eucaryotic proteins, when originally synthesized in the ribosome, start with a methionine. It is a kind of "start" signal in the genetic code. This methionine is generally re- moved before the protein is released into the cell, however. *Histidine* is a relatively rare amino acid, but often appears in the *active site* of an enzyme. The active site is the small portion of an enzyme that effects the target reaction, and it is the key to understanding the chemistry involved. The rest of the enzyme provides the necessary scaffolding to bring the active site to bear in the right place, and to keep it away from bonds that it might do harm to. Other regions of enzymes can also act as a switch, turning the active site on and off in a process called *allosteric* control. Because histidine's pK is near the typical pH of a cell, it is possible for small, local changes in the chemical environment to flip it back and forth between being charged and not charged. This ability to flip between states makes it useful for catalyzing chemical reactions. Other charged residues also sometimes play a similar role in catalysis (8). With this background, it is now possible to understand the basics of the protein folding problem. The genetic code specifies only the amino acid sequence of a protein. As a new protein comes off the ribosome, it folds up into the shape that gives it its biochemical function, sometimes called its *active conformation* (the same protein unfolded into some other shape is said to be *denatured*, which is what happens, *e.g.* to the white of an egg when you cook it). In the cell, this process takes a few seconds, which is a very long time for a chemical reaction. The complex structure of the ribosome may play a role in protein folding, and a few proteins need helper molecules, termed *chaperones* to fold properly. However, these few seconds are a very short time compared to how long it takes people to figure out how a protein will fold. In raw terms, the folding problem involves finding the mapping from primary sequence (a sequence of from dozens to several thousand symbols, drawn from a 20 letter alphabet) to the real-numbered locations of the thousands of constituent atoms in three space. Although all of the above features of amino acids play some role in protein folding, there are few absolute rules. The conformation a protein finally assumes will minimize the total "free" energy of the molecule. Going against the tendencies described above (*e.g.* packing several large sidechains near each other) increases the local free energy, but may reduce the energy elsewhere in the molecule. Each one of the tendencies described can be traded off against some other contribution to the total free energy of the folded protein. Given any conformation of atoms, it is possible in principle to compute its free energy. Ideally, one could examine all the possible conformations of a protein, calculate the free energy by applying quantum mechanical rules, and select the minimum energy conformation as a prediction of the folded structure. Unfortunately, there are very many possible conformations to test, and each energy calculation itself is prohibitively complex. A wide variety of approaches have been taken to making this problem tractable, and, given a few hours of super- computer time, it is currently possible to evaluate several thousand possible conformations. These techniques are well surveyed in Karplus & Petsko (11). An alternative to the pure physical simulations are the various approaches which a significant portion of this volume is dedicated to describing. The position of the atoms in a folded protein is called its *tertiary* structure. The *primary* structure is the amino acid sequence. *Secondary* structure refers to local arrangements of a few to a few dozen amino acid residues take on particular conformations that are seen repeatedly in many different proteins. These shapes are stabilized by *hydrogen bonds* (a hydrogen bond relatively weak bond that also plays a role in holding the two strands DNA molecule together). There are two main kinds of secondary structure: corkscrew-shaped conformations where the amino acids are packed together, called α-*helices*, and long flat sheets made up of two or more adjacent strands of the molecule, extended so that the amino acids are stretched out as far from each other as they can be. Each extended chain is called *strand*, and two or more β -strands held together by hydrogen bonds called a β-*sheet*. β -sheets can be composed of strands running in the same direction (called a *parallel* β -sheet) or running in the opposite direction *antiparallel*). Other kinds of secondary structure include structures that even more tightly packed than β -helices called *3-10 helices*, and a variety small structures that link other structures, called β *-turns*. Some local combinations of secondary structures have been observed in a variety of different proteins. For example, two α -helices linked by a turn with an approximately 60° angle have been observed in a variety of proteins that bind to DNA. pattern is called the *helix-turn-helix* motif, and is an example of what known as *super-secondary* structure. Finally, some proteins only become functional when assembled with other molecules. Some proteins bind copies of themselves; for example, some DNA-binding proteins only function as dimers (linked pairs). Other proteins require prostehtic groups such heme or chlorophyl. Additions necessary to make the folded protein are termed the protein's *quaternary* structure.

Nucleic Acids

If proteins are the workhorses of the biochemical world, nucleic acids their drivers; they control the action. All of the genetic information living creature is stored in deoxyribonucleic acid (DNA) and ribonucleic (RNA), which are polymers of four simple nucleic acid units, called *nucleotides*. There are four nucleotides found in DNA. Each nucleotide consists of three parts: one of two base molecules (a *purine* or a *pyrimidine*), sugar (ribose in RNA and deoxyribose DNA), and one or more phosphate groups. The purine nucleotides are *adenine* (A) and *guanine* (G), and pyrimidines are *cytosine* (C) and *thymine* (T). Nucleotides are sometimes called bases, and, since DNA consists of two complementary strands bonded together, these units are often called base-pairs. The length of a DNA sequences is often measured in thousands of bases, abbreviated kb. Nucleotides are generally abbreviated by their first letter, and appended into sequences, written, *e.g.*, CCTATAG. The nucleotides are linked to each other in the polymer by phosphodiester bonds. This bond is directional, a strand of DNA has a head (called the *5′* end) and a tail (the *3′* end). One well known fact about DNA is that it forms a double helix; that is, two *helical* (spiral-shaped) strands of the polypeptide, running in opposite directions, held together by hydrogen bonds. Adenines bond exclusively with the thymines (A-T) and guanines bond exclusively with cytosines (G-C). Although the sequence in one strand of DNA is completely unrestricted, because of these bonding rules the sequence in the complementary strand completely determined. It is this feature that makes it possible to make high fidelity copies of the information stored in the DNA. It is also exploited when DNA is transcribed into complementary strands of RNA, which direct the synthesis of protein. The only difference is that in RNA, uracil (U) takes the place of thymine; that is, it bonds to adenine. DNA molecules take a variety of conformations (shapes) in living systems. In most biological circumstances, the DNA forms a classic double helix, called B-DNA; in certain circumstances, however, it can become supercoiled or even reverse the direction of its twist (this form is called ZDNA). These alternative forms may play a role in turning particular genes on and off. There is some evidence that the geometry of the B-DNA form (e.g for example, differing twist angles between adjacent base pairs) may also be exploited by cell mechanisms. Now that we have described the basic structure and function of proteins and nucleic acids, we can begin to put together a picture of the molecular processing that goes on in every cell.

Genetic Expression: From Blueprint to Finished Product

Genes, the Genome and the Genetic Code

The genetic information of an organism can be stored in one or more distinct DNA molecules; each is called a *chromosome*. In some sexually reproducing organisms, called *diploids*, each chromosome contains two similar DNA molecules physically bound together, one from each parent. Sexually reproducing organisms with single DNA molecules in their chromosomes are called haploid. Human beings are diploid with 23 pairs of linear chromosomes. In Bacteria, it is common for the ends of the DNA molecule to bind together, forming a circular chromosome. All of the genetic information of an organism, taken together as a whole, is refered to as its *genome*. The primary role of nucleic acids is to carry the encoding of the primary structure of proteins. Each non-overlapping triplet of nucleotides, called a *codon*, corresponds to a particular amino acid (table 1). Four nucleotides can form $4^3 = 64$ possible triplets, which is more than the 20 needed to code for each amino acid (pairs would provide only 16 codons). Three of these codons are used to designate the end of a protein sequence, and are called stop codons. The others all code for a particular amino acid. That means that most amino acids are encoded by more than one codon. For example, alanine is represented in DNA by the codons GCT, GCC, GCA and GCG. Notice that the first two nucleotides of these codons are all identical, and that the third is redundant. Although this is not true for all of the amino acids, most codon synonyms differ only in the last nucleotide. This phenomenon is called the *degeneracy* of the code. Whether it is an artifact of the evolution, or serves a purpose such as allowing general changes in the global composition of DNA (*e.g.* increasing the proportion of purines) without changing the coded amino acids is still unknown. There are some small variations in the translation of codons into amino acids from organism to organism. Since the code is so central to the functioning of the cell, it is very strongly conserved over evolution. However, there are a few systems that use a slightly different code. An important example is found in mitochondria. Mitochondria have their own DNA, and probably represent previously free living organisms that were enveloped by eucaryotes. Mitochondrial DNA is translated using a slightly different code, which is more degenerate (has less information in the third nucleotide) than the standard code. Other organisms that diverged very early in evolution, such as the ciliates, also use different codes. The basic process of synthesizing proteins maps from a sequence of codons to a sequence of amino acids. However, there are a variety of important complications. Since codons come in triples, there are three possible places to start parsing a segment of DNA. For example, the chain...AATGCGATAAG... could be read...AAT-GCG-ATA... or...ATG-CGATAA... or...TGC-GAT-AAG.... Each of these parsings is called a *reading frame*. A parsing with a long enough string of codons with no intervening stop codons is called an *open reading frame*, or *ORF*; and could be translated into a protein. Organisms sometimes code different proteins with overlapping reading frames, so that if the reading process shifts by one character, a completely different, but still functional protein results! More often, frame shifts, which can be introduced by insertions and deletions in the DNA se- quence or transcriptional "stuttering," produce nonsense. Not only are there three possible reading frames in a DNA sequence, it is possible to read off either strand of the double helix. Recall that the second strand is the complement of the first, so that our example above (AATGCGATAAG) can also be read inverted and in the opposite direction, *e.g.* CTTATCGCATT. This is sometimes called reading from the *antisense* or *complementary* strand. An antisense message can also be parsed three ways, making a total of 6 possible reading frames for every DNA sequence. There are known examples of DNA sequences that code for proteins in both directions with several overlapping reading frames: quite a feat of compact encoding. And there's more. DNA sequences coding for a single protein in most eucaryotes have noncoding sequences, called *introns*, inserted into them. These introns are spliced out before the sequence is mapped into amino acids. Different eucaryotes have a variety of different systems for recognizing and removing these introns. Most bacteria don't have introns. It is not known whether introns evolved only after the origin of eucaryotes, or whether selective pressure has caused bacteria to lose theirs. The segments of DNA that actually end up coding for a protein are called *exons*. You can keep these straight by remembering that introns are insertions, and that exons are expressed. DNA contains a large amount of information in addition to the coding sequences of proteins. Every cell in the body has the same DNA, but each cell type has to generate a different set of proteins, and even within a single cell type, its needs change throughout its life. An increasing number of DNA signals that appear to play a role in the control of expression are being characterized. There are a variety of signals identifying where proteins begin and end, where splices should occur, and an exquisitely detailed set of mechanisms for controlling which proteins should be synthesized and in what quantities. DNA is sometimes found in single strands, particularly in some viruses. Viruses also play other tricks with nucleic acids, such as transcribing RNA into DNA, going against the normal flow of information in the cell. Even non-standard base-pairings sometimes play an important role, such as in the structure of transfer RNA (5).

RNA: Transcription, Translation, Splicing and RNA Structure

The process of mapping from DNA sequence to folded protein in eucaryotes involves many steps. The first step is the *transcription* of a portion of DNA into an RNA molecule, called a messenger RNA (mRNA). This process begins with the binding of a molecule called RNA polymerase to a location on the DNA molecule. Exactly where that polymerase binds determines which strand of the DNA will be read and in which direction. The DNA near the beginning of a protein coding region contain signals which can be recognized by the polymerase; (these regions) are called *promoters*. Polymerase catalyzes a reaction which causes the DNA to be used as a template to create a complementary strand of RNA, called the *primary transcript*. This transcript contains introns as well as exons. At the end of transcript, 250 or more extra adenosines, called a *poly-A tail*, are often to the RNA. The role of these nucleotides is not known, but the distinctive signature is sometimes used to detect the presence of mRNAs. The next step is the *splicing* the exons together. This operation takes place in a ribosome-like assembly called a *spliceosome*. The RNA remaining after the introns have been spliced out is called a *mature* mRNA, is then transported out of the nucleus to the cytoplasm, where it then to a ribosome. A ribosome is a very complex combination of RNA and protein, and operation has yet to be completely understood. It is at the ribosome that mRNA is used as a blueprint for the production of a protein; this process called *translation*. The reading frame that the translation will use is determined by the ribosome. The translation process depends on the presence molecules which make the mapping from codons in the mRNA to amino acids; these molecules are called *transfer-RNA* or *tRNAs*. tRNAs have anti-codon (that binds to its corresponding codon) near one end and the corresponding amino acid on the other end. The anti-codon end of the tRNAs bind to the mRNA, bringing the amino acids corresponding the mRNA sequence into physical proximity, where they form peptide bonds with other. How the tRNAs find only the correct amino acid was a mystery quite recently. This process depends on the three dimensional structure RNA molecule. As protein comes off the ribosome, it folds up into its native conformation. The process may involve help from the ribosome itself or from chaperone molecules, as was described above. Once the protein has folded, other transformations can occur. Various kinds of chemical groups can be bound to different places on the proteins, including sugars, phosphate, actyl or methyl groups. These additions change the hyrogen bonding proclivity or shape of the protein, and may necessary to make the protein active, or may keep it from having an before it is needed. The general term for these transformations is *post-translational modifications*. Once this process is complete, the protein is transported to the part of the cell where it will accomplish its function. Transport process may be merely passive diffusion through the cytoplasm, there may be an active transport mechanism that moves the protein across membranes or into the appropriate cellular compartment.

Genetic Regulation

Every cell has the same DNA. Yet the DNA in some cells codes for the proteins needed to function as, say, a muscle, and other code for the proteins make the lens of the eye. The difference lies in the regulation of the genetic machinery. At any particular time, a particular cell is producing only a small fraction of the proteins coded for in its DNA. And the amount of each protein produced must be precisely regulated in order for the cell to function properly. The cell will change the proteins it synthesizes in response to environment or other cues. The mechanisms that regulate this process constitute a finely tuned, highly parallel system with extensive multifactoral feedback and elaborate control structure. It is also not yet well understood. Genes are generally said to be on or off (or *expressed/not expressed*), although the amount of protein produced is also important. The production process is controlled by a complex collection of proteins in the nucleus eucaryotic cells that influence which genes are expressed. Perhaps the important of these proteins are the *histones*, which are tightly bound to DNA in the chromosomes of eucaryotes. Histones are some of the most conserved proteins in all of life. There are almost no differences in the sequence of plant and mammalian histones, despite more than a billion years of divergence in their evolution. Other proteins swarm around the DNA, some influencing the production of a single gene (either encouraging or inhibiting it), while others can influence the production of large numbers of genes once. An important group of these proteins are called *topoisomerases*; rearrange and untangle the DNA in various ways, and are the next prevalent proteins in the chromosome. Many regulatory proteins recognize and bind to very specific sequences the DNA. The sequences that these proteins recognize tend to border the protein coding regions of genes, and are known generally as *control regions*. Sequences that occur just upstream (towards the 5' end) of the coding region that encourage the production of the protein are called *promoters*. Similar regions either downstream of the coding

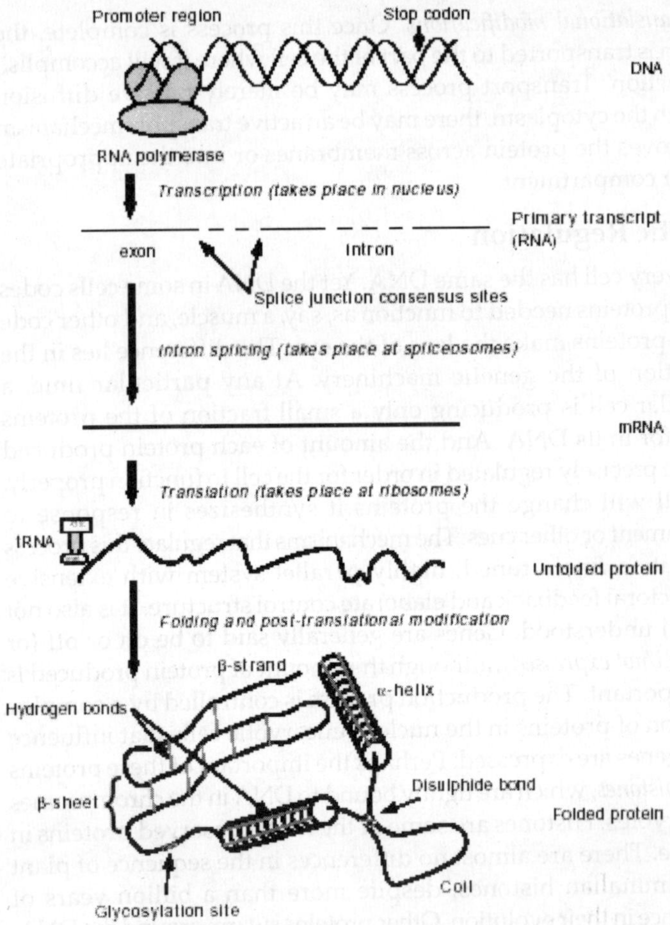

Figure 1.2: A Schematic Drawing of the Entire Process of Protein Synthesis. [An RNA Polymerase binds to a promoter region of DNA, and begins the transcription process,which continues until a stop codon is reached.The product is an RNA molecule called the primary transcript, which contains regions that code for proteins (exons) and regions which do not (introns). The introns are spliced out at splicosomes, and the joined exons are transported to a ribosome. There, transfer RNAs match amino acids to the appropriate codons in the RNA; the amino acids form peptide bonds and become an unfolded protein. The protein then folds into local formations like helices and sheets, and forms internal bonds across longer distances. Post-translational processing can add additional substance; e.g., glycosylation adds sugar molecules to the protein.]

region or relatively far upstream called *enhancers.* Sequences that tend to prevent the production of a protein are called *repressors.* Cells need to turn entire suites of genes on and off in response to many different events, ranging from normal development to trying to repair damage to the cell. The control mechanisms are responsive to the level of a product already in the cell (for homeostatic control) as well as to a tremendous variety of extracellular signals. Perhaps the most amazing activities in regulation occur during development; not only are genes turned on and with precise timing, but the control can extend to producing alternative splicings of the nascent primary transcripts (as is the case in the transition from fetal to normal hemoglobin).

Catalysis and Metabolic Pathways

The translation of genes into proteins, crucial as it is, is only a small portion of the biochemical activity in a cell. Proteins do most of the work of managing the flow of energy, synthesizing, degrading and transporting materials, sending and receiving signals, exerting forces on the world, and providing structural support. Systems of interacting proteins form the basis for nearly every process of living things, from moving around and digesting food to thinking and reproducing. Somewhat surprisingly, a large proportion of the chemical processes that underlie all of these activities are shared across a very wide range of organisms. These shared processes are collectively referred to as *intermediary metabolism.* These include the *catabolic* processes for breaking down proteins, fats and carbohydrates (such as those found in food) and the *anabolic* processes for building new materials. Similar collections of reactions that are more specialized to particular organisms are called *secondary metabolism.* The substances that these reactions produce and consume are called *metabolites.* The biochemical processes in intermediary metabolism are almost all *catalyzed reactions.* That is, these reactions would barely take place at all at normal temperatures and pressures; they require special compounds that facilitate the reaction–these compounds are called *catalysts* or *enzymes.* Catalysts are usually named after the reaction they facilitate, usually with the added suffix. For example, alcohol dehydrogenase is the enzyme that turns ethyl alcohol into acetaldehyde by removing two hydrogen atoms. Common classes of enzymes include *dehydrogenases, synthetases, proteases* (for breaking down proteins), *decarboxylases* (removing carbon atoms), *transferases* (moving a chemical group from one place to another), *kinases, phosphatases* (adding or removing phosphate groups, respectively) and so on. The materials transformed by catalysts are called *substrates.* Unlike the substrates, catalysts themselves are not changed by the reactions they participate in. A final point to note about enzymatic reactions is that in many cases the reactions can proceed in either direction. That is, and enzyme that transforms substance A into substance B can often also facilitate the transformation of B into A. The direction of the transformation depends on the concentrations of the substrates and on the energetics of the reaction. Even the basic transformations of intermediary metabolism can involve dozens or hundreds of catalyzed reactions. These combinations of reactions, which accomplish tasks like turning foods into useable energy or compounds are called metabolic *pathways.* Because of the many steps in these pathways and the widespread presence of direct and indirect feedback loops, they can exhibit many counterintuitive behaviors. Also, all of these chemical reactions are going on in parallel. In addition to the feedback loops among the substrates in the pathways, the presence or absence of substrates can affect the behavior of the enzymes themselves, through what is called *allosteric* regulation. These interactions occur when a substance binds to an enzyme someplace other than its usual *active site* (the atoms in the molecule that have the enzymatic effect). Binding at this other site changes the shape of the enzyme, thereby changing its activity. Another method of controlling enzymes is called *competitive inhibition.* In this form of regulation, substance other than the usual substrate of the enzyme binds to the active site of the enzyme, preventing it from having an effect on its substrate. These are the basic mechanisms underlying eucaryotic cells (and much of this applies to bacterial and archaeal ones as well). Of course, each particular activity of a living system, from the capture of energy to immune response, has its own complex network of biochemical reactions that provides the mechanism underlying the function. Some of these mechanisms, such as the *secondary messenger system* involving cyclic adenosine monophosphate cAMP) are widely shared by many different systems.

Genetic Mechanisms of Evolution and Mutation

The mechanisms of evolution at the molecular level are increasingly well understood (16). The similarities and differences among molecules that are closely related provide important information about the structure and function of those molecules. Molecules (or their sequences) which are related to one another are said to be *homologous.* Although genes or proteins that have similar sequences are often assumed to be homologous, there are well known counter examples due to *convergent evolution* (3).

In these cases, aspects of very distantly related organisms come to resemble one another through very different evolutionary pathways. Unless there is evidence to the contrary, it is usually safe to assume that macromolecular sequences that are similar to each other are homologous. The sources of variation at the molecular level are very important to understanding how molecules come to differ from each other (or *diverge).* Perhaps the best known mechanism of molecular evolution is the *point mutation,* or the change of a single nucleotide in a genetic sequence. The change can be to *insert* a new nucleotide, to *delete* an existing one, or to change one nucleotide into another. Other mechanisms include large scale chromosomal rearrangements and inversions. An important kind of rearrangement is the *gene duplication;* in which additional copies of a gene are inserted into the genome. These copies can then diverge, so that, for example, the original functionality may be preserved at the same time as related new genes evolve. These duplication events can lead to the presence of *pseudogenes,* which are quite similar to actual genes, but are not expressed. Sexual reproduction adds another dimension to the exchange of genetic material. DNA from the two parents of a sexually reproducing organism undergoes a process called *crossover,* which forms a kind of mosaic that is passed on to the offspring (17).

Most mutations have relatively little effect. Mutations in the middle of introns generally have no effect at all (although mutations at the ends of an intron can affect the splicing process). Mutations in the third position of most codons have little effect at the protein level because of the redundancy of the genetic code. Even mutations that cause changes in the sequence of a protein are often neutral, as demonstrated by Sauer, *et al* (22). Their experimental method involved *saturation mutagenesis* which explores are relatively large proportion of the space of possible mutations in parallel. Neutral mutations are the basis of genetic drift, which is the phenomena that accounts for the differences between the DNA that codes for functionally identical proteins in different organisms. This drift is also the basis for the molecular clock. Of course, some point mutations are lethal, and others lead to diseases such as cystic fibrosis. Very rarely, a mutation will be advantageous; it will then rapidly get fixed in the population, as the organisms with the conferred advantage out reproduce the ones without it. Diploid sexually reproducing organisms have two copies of each gene (one from each parent), resulting in an added layer of complexity in the effect of mutations. Sometimes the extra copy can compensate (or partially compensate) for a mutation.

Molecular evolution also involves issues of selection and inheritance. Inheritance requires that the genes from the parent be passed to the offspring. DNA itself is replicated by splitting the double helix into two complimentary strands and then extending a primer by attaching complementary nucleotides. The molecular mechanisms underlying the whole complex process of cell division (*i.e.* the cell cycle) are strikingly conserved in eucaryotes, and knowledge about this process is growing rapidly (Hartwell (9)). Selection also occurs on factors that are only apparent on the molecular level, such as the efficiency of certain reaction pathways (Hochachka & Somero, (10)).

Model Organisms

The investigation of the workings of even a single organism is so complex as to take many dedicated scientists many careers worth of time. Trying to study all organisms in great depth is simply beyond the abilities of modern biology. Furthermore, the techniques of biological experimentation are often complex, time consuming and difficult. Some of the most valuable methods in biological research are invasive, or require organisms to be sacrificed, or require many generations of observation, or observations on large populations. Much of this work is impractical or unethical to carry out on humans.

For these reasons, biologists have selected a variety of model organisms for experimentation. These creatures have qualities that make possible controlled laboratory experiments at reasonable cost and difficulty with results that can often be extrapolated to people or other organisms of interest. Of course, research involving humans can be done ethically, and in some areas of biomedical research, such as final drug testing, it is obligatory. Other research methods involve kinds of human cells can be grown successfully in the laboratory. Not many human cell types thrive outside of the body (4). Some kinds of human cancer cells do grow well in the laboratory, and these cells are an important vehicle for research. Sometimes the selection of a new model organism can lead to great advances in a field. For example, the use of a particular kind of squid made possible the understanding of the functioning of neurons because it contained motor neuron that is more than 10 times the size of most neural cells, and hence easy to find and use in experiments. There are experimentally useful correlates of nearly every aspect of human biology found in some organism or another, but the following six organisms form the main collection of models used in molecular biology (18-20).

E. coli

The ubiquitous intestinal bacterium *Escherichia coli* is a workhorse in biological laboratories. Because it is a relatively simple organism with fast reproduction time and is safe and easy to work with, *E. coli* has been the focus of a great deal of research in genetics and molecular biology of the cell. Although it is a Bacterium, many of the basic biochemical mechanisms of *E. coli* are shared by humans. For example, the first understanding of how genes can be turned on and off came from the study of a virus that infects these bacteria (Ptashne, (21)). *E. coli* is a common target for genetic engineering, where genes from other organisms are inserted into the bacterial genome then produced in quantity. *E. coli* is now the basis of the international biotechnology industry, churning out buckets full of human insulin, the heart attack drug TPA, and a wide variety of other substances.

Saccharomyces cervesiae

This is better known as brewer's yeast, and it is another safe, easy to grow, short generation time organism.

Other yeasts, such as *Schizosaccharomyces pombe*, are also used extensively. Surprisingly, yeasts are very much like people in many ways. Unlike the bacterium *E. coli*, yeasts are eucaryotes, with a cell nucleus, mitochondria, a eucaryotic cell membrane, and many of the other cellular components and processes found in most other eucaryotes, including people. Because these yeasts are so easy to grow and manipulate, and because they are so biochemically similar to people, many insights about the molecular processes involved in metabolism, biosynthesis, cell division, and other crucial areas of biology have come from the investigation of *Saccharomyces* (Saccharomyces is a genus name, which, when used alone, refers to all species that are within that genus). Yeasts play another important role in molecular biology. One of the crucial steps in sequencing large amounts of DNA is to be able to prepare many copies of moderate sized pieces of DNA.

Arabidopsis

The most important application of increased biological understanding is generally thought to be in medicine, and increased understanding of human biology has indeed led to dramatic improvements in health care. However, in terms of effect on human life, agriculture is just as significant. A great deal of research into genetics and biochemistry has been motivated by the desire to better understand various aspects of plant biology. An important model organism for plants is *Arabidopsis thaliana*, a common weed. *Arabidopsis* makes a good model because it undergoes the same processes of growth, development, flowering and reproduction as most higher plants, but it's genome has 30 times less DNA than corn, and very little repetitive DNA.It also produces lots of seeds, and takes only about six weeks to grow to maturity. There are several other model organisms used to investigate botanical questions, including tomatoes, tobacco, carrots and corn.

Caenorhabditis

One of the most exciting model organisms to emerge recently has been the nematode worm *Caenorhabditis elegans.* This tiny creature, thousands of which can be found in a spadeful of dirt, has already been used to generate tremendous insight about cellular development and physiology. Every normal worm consists of exactly the same collection of cells in the same places doing the same thing.It is one of the simplest creatures with a nervous system. Not only is the complete anatomy of the organism known, but also a complete cell fate map has been generated, tracing the developmental lineage of each of each cell throughout the lifespan of the organism. This map allows researchers to relate behaviors to particular cells, to trace the effects of genetic mutations very specifically, and perhaps to gain insight into the mechanisms of aging as well as development. A large, highly integrated picture and text database of information about the cell fates, genetic maps and sequences, mutation effects and other relevant information about *C. elegans* is currently under construction at the University of Arizona.

Drosophila

Drosophila melanogaster common fruit fly, has long been a staple of classical genetics research. These flies have short generation times, and many different genetically determined morphological characteristics (*e.g.* eye color) that can readily be determined by visual inspection.

Drosophila were used for decades in exploring patterns of inheritance; now that molecular methods can be applied, they have proven invaluable for a variety of studies of genetic expression and control. An important class of genetic elements that regulate many other genes, in effect, specifying complex genetic programs, were first discovered in *Drosophila;* these areas are called *homeoboxes.* Molecular genetics in *Drosophila* is also providing great insights into how complex body plans are generated.

In Molecular biology in zebra fish is also providing great insights.

Mus

Mus musculus is the basic laboratory mouse. Mice are mammals, and, as far as biochemistry is concerned, are practically identical to people. Many questions about physiology, reproduction, functioning of the immune and nervous systems and other areas of interest can only be addressed by examining creatures that are very similar to humans; mice nearly always fit the bill. The similarities between mice and people mean also that the mouse is a very complicated creature; it has a relatively large, complex genome, and mouse development and physiology is not as regular or consistent as that of *C. elegans* or *Drosophila.* Although our depth of understanding of the mouse will lag behind understanding of simpler organisms, the comparison of mouse genome to human is likely to be a key step, both in understanding their vast commonalities, and in seeing the aspects of our genes that make us uniquely human.

Experimental Methods

Molecular biologists have developed a tremendous variety of tools to address questions of biological function.

Imaging

The first understanding of the cellular nature of life came shortly after the invention of the light microscope, and microscopy remaines central to research in biology The tools for creating images have expanded tremendously. Not only are there computer controled light microscopes with a wide variety of imaging modalities, but there are now many other methods of generating images of the very small. The electon microscope offers extremely high resolution, although it requires exposing the imaged sample to high vacuum and other harsh treatments. New technologies including the Atomic Force Microscope (AFM) and the Scanning Tunnelling Microscope (STM) offer the potential to create images of individual molecules. Biologists use these tools extensively (12).

Gel Electrophoresis

A charged molecule, when placed in an electric field, will be accelerated; positively charged molecules will move toward negative electrodes and vice versa. By placing a mixture of molecules of interest in a medium and subjecting them to an electric charge, the molecules will migrate through the medium and separate from each other. How fast the molecules will move depends on their charge and their size-bigger molecules see more resistance from the medium. The procedure, called *electrophoresis* involves putting a spot of the mixture to be analyzed at the top of a polyacrylamide or agarose gel, and applying an electric field for a period of time. Then the gel is stained so that the molecules become visible; the stains appear as stripes along the gel, and are called *bands.* The location of the bands on the gel are proportional to the charge and size of the molecules in the mixture. The intensity of the stain is an indication of the amount of a particular molecule in the mixture. If the molecules are all the same charge, or have charge proportional to their size (as, for example, DNA does) then electrophoresis separates them purely by size.

Often, several mixtures are run simultaneously on a single gel. This allows for easy calibration to standards, or comparison of the contents of different mixtures, showing, for example, the absence of a particular molecular component in one. The adjacent, parallel runs are sometimes called *lanes*. A variation on this technique allows the sorting of molecules by a chemical property called the *isoelectric point*, which is related to its pK. A combination of the two methods, called

2D electrophoresis is capable of very fine distinctions, for example, mapping each protein in a cell to a unique *spot* in two-space, the size of the spot indicating the amount of the protein. Although there are still some difficulties in calibration and repeatability, this method is potentially a very powerful tool for monitoring the activities of large biochemical systems. In addition, if a desired molecule can be separated from the mixture this way, individual spots or bands can be removed from the gel for further processing, in a procedure called *blotting*.

Cloning

A group of cells with identical genomes are said to be *clones* of one another. Unless there are mutations, a single cell that reproduces asexually will produce identical offspring; these clones are sometimes called a *cell line*, and certain standardized cell lines, for example the HeLa cell line, play an important role in biological research.

This concept has been generalize to cloning individual genes. In this case, a piece of DNA containing a gene of interest is inserted into the genome of a target cell line, and the cells are screened so that all of the resulting cells have an identical copy of the desired genetic sequence. The DNA in these cells is said to be *recombinant*, and the cell will produce the protein coded for by the inserted gene. Cloning a gene requires some sophisticated technology. In order for a cloned gene to be expressed, it must contain the appropriate transcription signals for the target cell line. One way biologists ensure that this will happen is to put the new gene into a bacteriophage (a virus that infects bacteria), or a plasmid (a circular piece of DNA found outside of the chromosome of bacteria that replicates independently of the bacteria's chromosomal DNA). These devices for inserting foreign DNA into cells are called *vectors*. In order to cut and paste desired DNA fragments into vectors, biologists use *restriction enzymes*, which cut DNA at precisely specified points. These enzymes are produced naturally by bacteria as a way of attacking foreign DNA. For example, the commonly used enzyme *EcoRI* (from *E. coli)* cuts DNA between the G and the A in the sequence GAATTC; these target sequences are called *restriction sites*. Everywhere a restriction site occurs in a DNA molecule treated with *EcoRI*, the DNA will be broken. Restriction enzymes play many roles in biology in addition to making gene cloning possible; a few others will be described below.

Both the insertion of the desired gene into the vector and the uptake of the vector by the target cells are effective only a fraction of the time. Fortunately, cells and vectors are small and it is relatively easy to grow a lot of them. The process is applied to a population of target cells, and then the resulting population is screened to identify the cells where the gene was successfully inserted. This can be difficult, so many vectors are designed to facilitate screening. One popular vector, *pBR322*, contains a naturally occurring transcription start signal and some antibiotic resistance genes, designed with conveniently placed restriction sites. If this vector is taken up by the target cells, it will confer resistance to certain antibiotics to them. By applying the anitbiotic to the whole colony, the researcher can kill all the cells that did not get the cloned gene. More sophisticated manipulations involving multiple antibiotic resistances and carefully placed restriction sites can also be used to ensure that the gene was correctly taken up by the vector. There are many variations on these techniques for inserting foreign genes. It is now possible to use simple bacteria to produce large amounts of almost any isolated protein, including, for example, human insulin. Although it is a more complex process, it is also possible to insert foreign genes into plants and animals, even people. A variety of efforts are underway to use these techniques to engineer organisms for agriculture, medicine and other applications. Not all of these applications are benign. One of the most successful early efforts was to increase the resistance of tobacco plants to pesticides, and there are clear military applications. On the other hand, these methods also promise new approaches to producing important rare biological compounds inexpensively (*e.g.* for novel cancer treatments or cleaning up toxic waste) and improving the nutritional value or hardiness of agricultural products. The entire field of genetic engineering is controversial, and there are a variety of controls on what experiments can be done and how they can be done. Hybridization and Immunological Staining. Biological compounds can show remarkable specificity, for example, binding very selectively only to one particular compound. This ability plays an important role in the laboratory, where researchers can identify the presence or absence of a particular molecule (or even a region of a molecule) in vanishingly small amounts. *Antibodies* are the molecules that the immune system uses to identify and fight off invaders. Antibodies are extremely specific, recognizing and binding to only one kind of molecule. Dyes can be attached to the antibody, forming a very specific system for identifying the presence (and possibly quantifying the amount) of a target molecule that is present in a system. There is a conceptually related method for identifying very specifically the presence of a particular nucleotide sequence in a macromolecule. The complement to a single-stranded DNA sequence will bind quite specifically to that sequence. One technique measures how similar two related DNA sequences are by testing how strongly the single-stranded versions of the molecules stick to each other, or *hybridize*. The more easily they come apart, the more differences there are between their sequences. It is also possible to attach a dye or other marker to a specific piece of DNA (called a *probe*) and then hybridize it to a longer strand of DNA. The location along the strand that is complementary to the probe will then be marked. There are many variations on hybridization and immunological staining that are customized to the needs of a particular experiment.

Gene Mapping and Sequencing

The Human Genome Project is the effort to produce a map and then the sequence of the human genome. The purpose of a genetic map is to identify the location and size of all of the genes of an organism on its chromosomes. This information is important for a variety of reasons. First, because crossover is an important component of inheritance in sexually reproducing organisms, genes that are near each other on the chromosome will tend to be inherited together. In fact, this forms the basis for *linkage analysis*, which is a technique that looks at the relationships between genes (or phenotypes) in large numbers of matings (in this context, often called *crosses*) to identify which genes tend to be inherited together, and are therefore likely to be near each other. Second, it is possible to clone genes of known locations, opening up a wide range of possible experimental manipulations. Finally, it is currently possible to determine the sequence of moderate size pieces of DNA, so if an important gene has been mapped, it is possible to find the sequence of that area, and discover the protein that is responsible for the genetic characteristic. This is especially important for understanding the basis of inherited diseases. The existence of several different kinds of restriction enzymes makes possible a molecular method of creating genetic maps. The application of each restriction enzyme (the process is called a *digest*) creates a different collection of *restriction fragments* (the cut up pieces of DNA). By using gel electrophoresis, it is possible to determine the size of these fragments. Using multiple enzymes, together and separately, results in sets of fragments which can be (partially) ordered with respect to each other, resulting in a genetic map. These *physical maps* divide a large piece of DNA (like a chromosome) into parts, and and there is an associated method for obtaining any desired part (13-15, 19).

Restriction fragment mapping becomes problematic when applied to large stretches of DNA, because the enzymes can produce many pieces of about the same size, making the map ambiguous. The use of different enzymes can help address this problem to a limited degree, but a variety of other techniques are now also used.

Being able to divide the genome into moderate sized chunks is a prerequisite to determining its sequence. Although there are several clever methods for determining the sequence of DNA molecule, all of them are limited to a resolution of well under a thousand basepairs at a time. In order to take this sequencing ability and determine the sequence of large pieces of DNA, many different overlapping chunks must be sequenced, and then these sequences must be assembled. In order to accomplish this task, it is necessary to break the DNA in an entire genome down into a set of more manageable sized pieces. The ordering of these pieces must be known (so they can be reassembled into a complete sequence), taken together the pieces must cover the entire genome, and the same set of pieces must be accessible to many different laboratories. This process is usually accomplished in several stages. The first stage generates relatively large pieces called *contigs*. Contigs are maintained in cloned cell lines so that they can be reproduced and distributed. Often, these pieces of DNA are made into *Yeast artificial chromosomes*, or *YACs*, which can hold up to about a million basepairs of sequence each, requiring on the order of 10,000 clones to adequately cover the entire human genome. Each of these is then broken down into sets of smaller pieces, often in the form of *cosmids*. A cosmid is a particular kind of bacteriophage (a virus that infects bacteria) that is capable of accepting inserts of 30,000 or so basepairs. The difficulties in generating and maintaining collections of clones that large have led to alternative technologies for large scale sequencing. One alternative involves a new technology based on the *polymerase chain reaction*, or *PCR*. This mechanism was revolutionary becauase it made it possible to rapidly produce huge amounts of a specific region of DNA, simply by knowing a little bit of the sequence around the desired region. PCR exponentially *amplifies* (makes copies of) a segment of a DNA molecule, given a unique pair of sequences that bracket the desired piece. First, short sequences of DNA (called *oligonucleotides*, or *oligos*) complementary to each of the bracketing sequences are synthesized. Creating short pieces of DNA with a specific sequence is routine technology. These pieces are called *primers.* Te primers, the target DNA and the enzyme DNA polymerase are then combined. The mixture is heated, so that the hydrogen bonds in the DNA break and the molecule splits into two single strands. When the mixture cools sufficiently, the primers bond to the regions around the area of interest, and the DNA polymerase replicates the DNA downstream of the primers. By using a heat resistant polymerase from an Archaea species that lives at high temperatures, it is possible to rapidly cycle this process, doubling the amount of desired segment of DNA each time. This technology makes possible the exponential amplification of entire DNA molecules or any specific region of DNA for which bracketing primers can be generated.

In order to use PCR for genome mapping and sequencing, a collection of unique (short) sequences spread throughout the genome must be identified for use as primers. The sequences must be unique in the genome so that the source of amplified DNA is unambiguous, and they have to be relatively short so that they are easy to synthesize. The sites in the genome that correspond to these sequences are called *sequence tagged sites* or *STSs.* The more STSs that are known, the finer grained the map of the genome they provide. Finding short, unique sequences even in 3×10^9 bp of DNA is not that difficult; a simple calculation shows that most sequences of length 16 or so can reasonably be expected to be unique in a genome of that size. An early goal of the Human Genome Project is to generate a list of STSs spaced at approximately 100kbp intervals over the entire human genome. If it is possible to find STSs that adequately cover the genome, it will not be necessary to build and maintain libraries of 10,000 YACs and ten times as many cosmids. Any region of DNA of interest can be identified by two STSs that bracket it. Instead of having to maintain large clone collections, these STSs can be stored in a database, and any researcher who needs a particular section of DNA can synthesize the appropriate primers and use PCR to produce many copies of just of that section.

Another issue that has been raised about the project to sequence the genome is the need to know the sequences of all of the introns and other noncoding regions of DNA. One way to address this issue is to target only coding regions for sequencing. The ability to find the sequences that a particular cell is using to produce proteins at a particular point in time is also useful in a variety of other areas as well. This information can be gleaned by gathering the mRNAs present in the cytoplasm of the cell, and sequencing them. Instead of sequencing the mRNAs directly, biologists use an enzyme called *reverse transcriptase* to make DNA molecules complementary to the mRNAs (called *cDNAs*) and then sequence that DNA. Using PCR and other technology, it is possible to capture at least portions of most of the mRNAs a cell is producing. By sequencing these cDNAs, researchers can focus their attention on just the parts of the genome that code for expressed proteins.

Large scale attempts to sequence at least part of all of the cDNAs that can be produced from brain tissue have resulted in partial sequences for more than 2500 new proteins in a very short period of time (1). These sequences called ESTs, for *expressed sequence tags* can be used as PCR primers for future, more detailed experiments. This work has created controversy because of the ensuing attempt by the National Institutes of Health to patent the EST sequences.

Crystallography and NMR. Until the relationship between protein sequence and structure is more fully understood, the sequences produced by genome projects will provide only part of the biochemical story. Additional information about protein structure is necessary to understand how the proteins function. This structural information is at the present primarily gathered by *X-ray crystallography*. In order to determine the structure of a protein in this manner, a very large, pure crystal of the protein must be grown (this process can take years, and may never succeed for certain proteins). Then the X-ray diffraction pattern of the crystal is measured, and this information can be used indirectly to determine the positions of the atoms in the molecule (23).

Because of the difficulties in crystallography, relatively few structures are known, but the number of new structures is growing exponentially, with a doubling time of a bit over two years.

A promising alternative to crystallography for determining protein structure is multi-dimensional *nuclear magnetic resonance*, or

NMR. Although this process does not require the crystallization of the protein, there are technical difficulties in analyzing the data associated with large molecules like proteins. Both crystallography and NMR techniques result in static protein structures, which are to some degree misleading. Proteins are flexible, and the patterns of their movement are likely to play an important role in their function. Although NMR has the potential to provide information about this facet of protein activity, there is very little data available currently.

Chapter 2

Body Proteins and Relative Protein Drugs

You've probably heard that proteins are important nutrients that help you build muscles. But they are much more than that. Proteins are the worker molecules that make possible every activity in your body. They circulate in your blood, seep from your tissues, and grow in long strands out of your head. Proteins are also the key components of biological materials ranging from silk fibers to elk antlers.

Proteins Are Made From Small Building Blocks

Proteins are like long necklaces with differently shaped beads. Each "bead" is a small molecule called an amino acid. There are 20 standard amino acids, each with its own shape, size, and properties.

Proteins contain from 50 to 5,000 amino acids hooked end-to-end in many combinations. Each protein has its own sequence of amino acids.

These amino acid chains do not remain straight and orderly. They twist and buckle, folding in upon themselves, the knobs of some amino acids nestling into grooves in others.

Only when the protein settles into its final shape does it become active. This process is complete almost immediately after proteins are made. Most proteins fold in less than a second, although the largest and most complex proteins may require several seconds to fold. Some proteins need help from other proteins, called "chaperones," to fold efficiently.

Proteins Fold Into Spirals and Sheets

When proteins fold, they don't randomly wad up into twisted masses. Often, short sections of proteins form recognizable shapes such as "alpha helices" or "beta sheets." Alpha helices are spiral shaped and beta sheets are pleated structures. Scientists devised a stylized method of representing proteins, called a ribbon diagram, that highlights helices and sheets. These organized sections of a protein pack together with each other- or with other, less organized sections- to form the final, folded protein.

Table 2.1: The Genetic Code Explains How Sets of Three Nucleotides Code for Amino Acids. This code is stored in DNA, then transferred to messenger RNA (mRNA), from which new proteins are synthesized. RNA (ribonucleic acid) is chemically very similar to DNA and also contains four chemical letters. But there is one major difference: where DNA uses thymine (T), mRNA uses uracil (U).

UUU phenylalanine	UCU serine	UAU tyrosine	UGU cysteine
UUC phenylalanine	UCC serine	UAC tyrosine	UGC cysteine
UUA leucine	UCA serine	UAA stop	UGA stop
UUG leucine	UCG serine	UAG stop	UGG tryptophan
CUU leucine	CCU proline	CAU histidine	CGU arginine
CUC leucine	CCC proline	CAC histidine	CGC arginine
CUA leucine	CCA proline	CAA glutamine	CGA arginine
CUG leucine	CCG proline	CAG glutamine	CGG arginine
AUU isoleucine	ACU threonine	AAU asparagine	AGU serine
AUC isoleucine	ACC threonine	AAC asparagine	AGC serine
AUA isoleucine	ACA threonine	AAA lysine	AGA arginine
AUG methionine (start)	ACG threonine	AAG lysine	AGG arginine
GUU valine	GCU alanine	GAU aspartic acid	GGU glycine
GUC valine	GCC alanine	GAC aspartic acid	GGC glycine
GUA valine	GCA alanine	GAA glutamic acid	GGA glycine
GUG valine	GCG alanine	GAG glutamic acid	GGG glycine

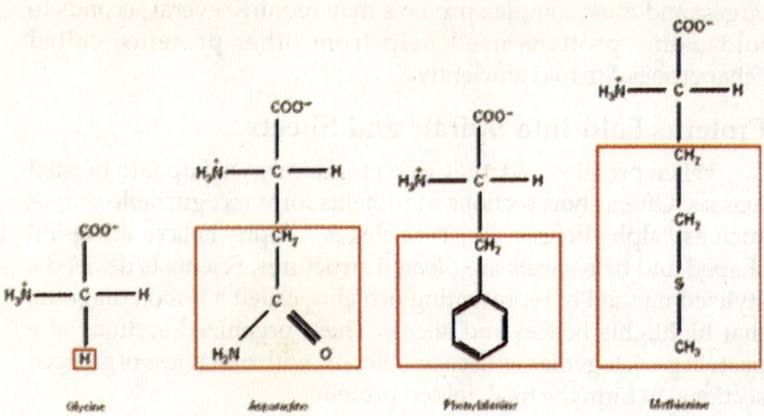

Fig. 2.1: Amino Acids are Like Differently Shaped "Beads" that Make Up Protein "Necklaces." (Shown here are a few examples of the 20 standard amino acids. Each amino acid contains an identical backbone structure (in black) and a unique side chain, also called an R-group (in red box). The shapes and chemical properties of these side chains are responsible for the twists and folds of the protein as well as for the protein's biological function.)

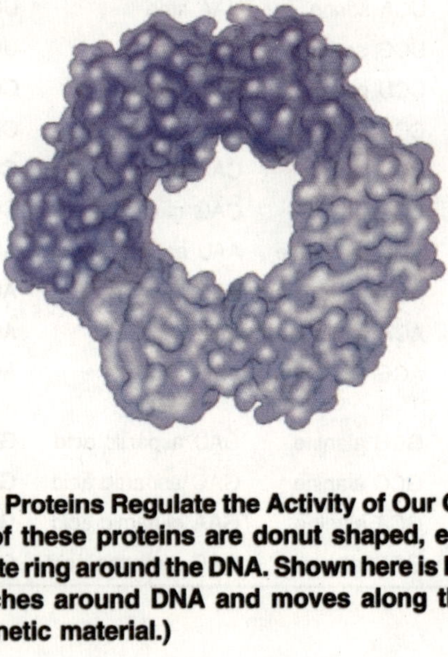

Fig. 2.2: Some Proteins Regulate the Activity of Our Genetic Material, DNA. (Some of these proteins are donut shaped, enabling them to form a complete ring around the DNA. Shown here is DNA polymerase III, which cinches around DNA and moves along the strands as it copies the genetic material.)

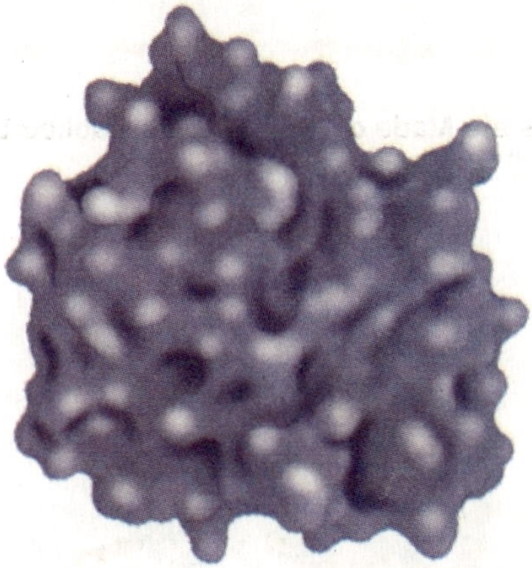

Fig. 2.3: Many Proteins, Like the Digestive Enzyme Chymotrypsin, are Somewhat Spherical in Shape. (Enzymes, which are proteins that facilitate chemical reactions, often contain a groove or pocket to hold the molecule they act upon.)

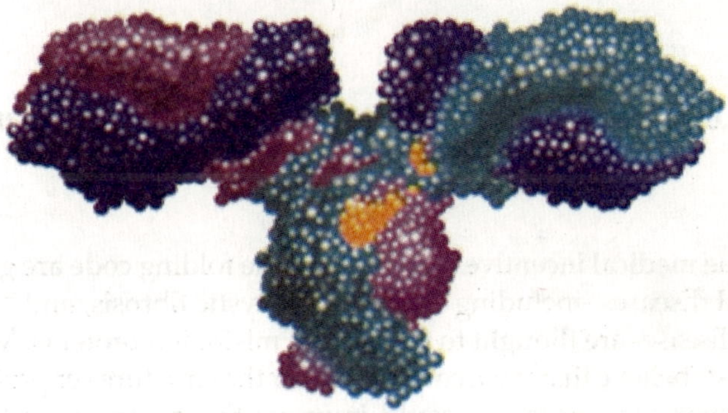

Fig. 2.4: Antibodies are Immune System Proteins that Rid the Body of Foreign Material, Including Bacteria and Viruses. (The two arms of the Y-shaped antibody bind to a foreign molecule. The stem of the antibody sends signals to recruit other members of the immune system.)

Scientists call this the "protein folding problem," and it remains one of the great challenges in structural biology. Although researchers have teased out some general rules and, in some cases, can make rough guesses of a protein's shape, they cannot accurately and reliably predict a final structure from an amino acid sequence (22).

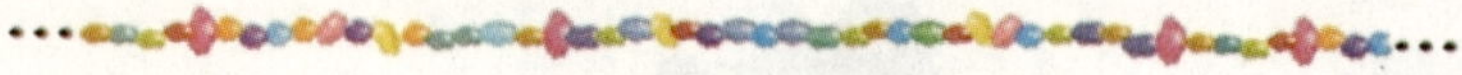

Fig. 2.5: Proteins are Made of Amino Acids Hooked End-to-end Like Beads on a Necklace.

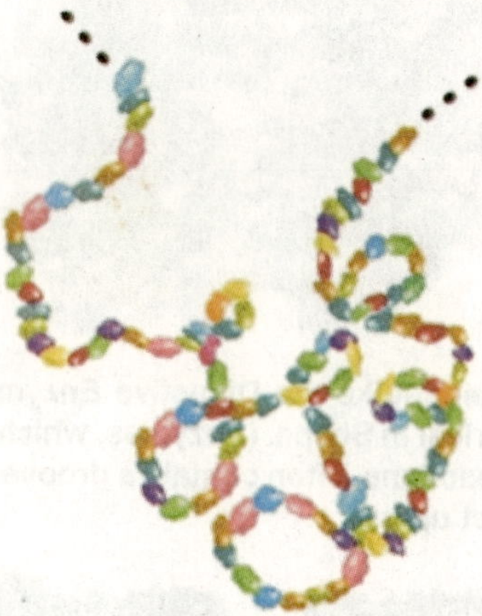

Fig. 2.6: To Become Active, Proteins Must Twist and Fold into their Final, or "Native," Conformation.

The medical incentives for cracking the folding code are great. Several diseases -including Alzheimer's, cystic fibrosis, and "mad cow" disease- are thought to result from misfolded proteins. Many scientists believe that if we could decipher the structures of proteins from their sequences, we could improve the treatment of these diseases.

Until recently, pharmaceuticals used for the treatment of diseases have been based largely on the production of relatively small organic molecules synthesized by microbes or by organic chemistry. These include most antibiotics, analgesics, hormones, and other pharmaceuticals. Increasingly, attention has focused on larger and more complex *protein* molecules as therapeutic agents. The structure and functionality of a given protein is determined by its sequence of amino acids, which, in turn, determines its three-dimensional conformation, or structure. Internal bonds (sulfur and hydrogen

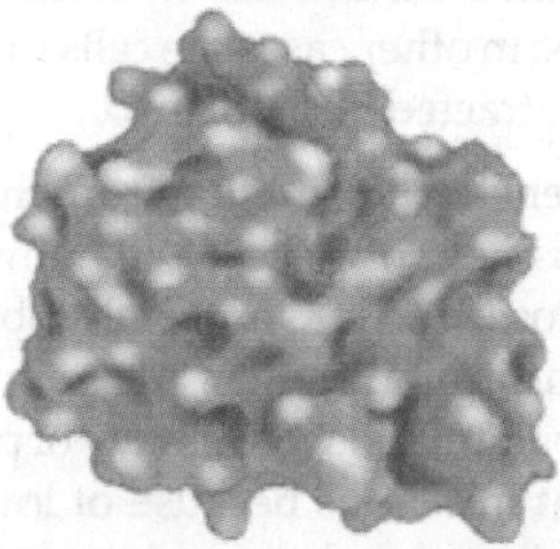

Fig. 2.7: This Final Shape Enables Proteins to Accomplish their Function in Your Body (Folded Protein).

bonds) among the amino acids give the protein its final shape and form. Complex proteins undergo further processing such as the addition of phosphate groups *(phosphorylation)* or carbohydrate molecules *(glycosylation)*, which modify the proteins' functions. Information stored in DNA directs the protein-synthesizing machinery of the cell to produce the specific proteins required for its structure and metabolism. Since proteins play critical roles in cell biology, they have many potential therapeutic uses in preventing and curing diseases and disorders. The first protein used to treat disease was insulin, a small *peptide* that revolutionized the treatment of diabetes. In addition, the *antigens* used in vaccinations to induce *immune responses* are often proteins. While short peptide chains (containing fewer than 30 amino acids) can be synthesized chemically, larger proteins are best produced by living cells. The DNA that encodes the instructions for producing the desired protein is inserted into cells, and as the cells grow they synthesize the protein, which is subsequently harvested and purified. Since 2003, more than 95 *therapeutic proteins*, or peptides *("biologics")*, have been licensed for production using bacterial, fungal, and mammalian cells grown in sterile cultures, and hundreds of additional therapeutic proteins are currently being developed and tested.

The pharmaceutical industry is undergoing remarkable changes with the discovery and introduction of biotech drugs. Biotech drugs are medicines that are therapeutic proteins. Today, there are more than 371 new biotechnology medicines in the pipeline. Cell cultures are grown in large stainless-steel fermentation vats under strictly maintained and regulated conditions. In some cases the proteins are secreted by the cells; in other cases the cells must be broken open so the protein can be extracted and purified.

The glut of new genetic information from the Human Genome Project is an embarrassment of riches. We know the sequences of thousands of genes whose functions are totally obscure. As sequence data accumulates, traditional means of assigning functions to unknown genes seem painfully slow. Delivery of protein therapeutics often requires frequent injections because of low activity or rapid clearance, thereby placing a burden on patients and caregivers.

Proteomics, a new technique for analyzing the proteins produced from the DNA in the cell promises to be of vital importance to the pharmaceutical industry in the development of new therapeutic drugs, the identification of mechanisms of drug resistance, and for solving a wide range of biological problems.

Chapter 3

Some Important Protein Based Drugs

Interferon (IFNs)

Interferon (IFNs) are naturally occurring glyco-protein in the body. They are produced only when required i.e when there is invasion from a foreign body such as Virus, Antigen or an inducer like formation of tumor etc. Interferon are originally produced by protein synthesis in the very small amount in the presence of the inducers (foreign bodies). Interferon are secreted by the cell into the extracellular fluids (Fig.)

There are mainly three types of **interferon–**

1. Alpha Interferon
2. Beta Interferon
3. Gamma Interferon

Differ in both ways structurally and antigenically and have molecular weights ranging from 16,000 to 45,000.

The interferon alpha (24 genes that code for Alpha) and beta Interferon (the single gene code for beta) in humans, are located in adjacent positions on chromosome 9.

The only gene for interferon gamma is found on chromosome

12. The genes for interferon alpha and beta exhibit significant homology but not with interferon gamma.

Types of Interferon

Alpha Interferon

- Contain 166 amino acids.
- At least 25 subtypes are present. Main sub types are **alpha 2a and alpha 2b**. Interferon-alpha-2a and interferon-alpha-2b are referred to as standard interferon.
- Mainly produced by leukocytes (white blood cells derived from bone marrow).
- It acts on type I receptor (multi-subunit receptor) of the cell.
- **Interferon alpha 2a** and **Interferon alpha 2b** are only structurally different but functionally they are same. The metabolism is also same in **Interferon alpha 2a** and **Interferon alpha 2b.**

Interferon Alpha 2a

- Following figure shows the structure of Interferon Alpha 2a

```
      SH
NH2-C D L P Q T H S L G   N R R A L I L L A Q
                    SH
    M G R I S P F S C L   K D R H D F G F P Q
    E E F D G N Q F Q K   A Q A I S V L H E M
    I Q Q T F N L F S T   K D S S A T W D E S
                                          SH
    L L E K F Y T E L Y   Q Q L N D L E A C V
    I Q E V G V E E T P   L M N E D S I L A V
    R K Y F Q R I T L Y   L T-COOH
```

- **Roferon-A** (produced by Roche Laboratories) is interferon-alpha-2a
- **Alferon** from Zydus.
- **Shanferon** from Shantha Biotech

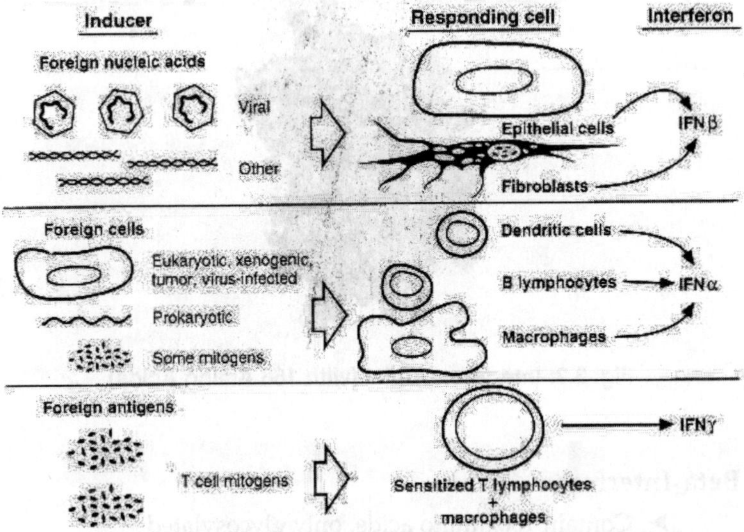

Fig. 3.1: Induction of Beta Interferon, Alpha Interferon, and Gamma Interferon, Respectively, by Foreign Nucleic Acids, Foreign Cells, and Foreign Antigens.

Interferon Alpha 2B

➤ Following figure shows the structure of Interferon Alpha 2B

```
     SH
NH2-C D L P Q T H S L G   N R R A L I L L A Q
                    SH
    M G R I S P F S C L   K D R H D F G F P Q

    E E F D G N Q F Q K   A Q A I S V L H E M

    I Q Q T F N L F S T   K D S S A T W D E S
                                          SH
    L L E K F Y T E L Y   Q Q L N D L E A C V

    I Q E V G V E E T P   L M N E D S I L A V

    R K Y F Q R I T L Y   L T-COOH
```

➤ **Mark-Feron** is interferon-alpha-2b.

➤ **Intron-A** (produced by Schering-Plough) is also interferon-alpha-2b.

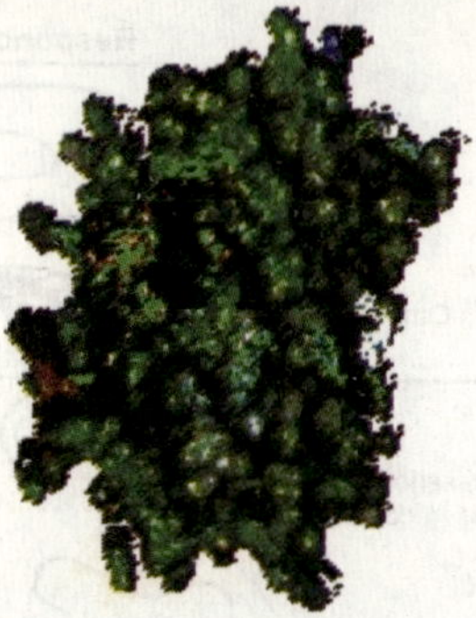

Fig. 3.2: Interferon Alpha (with 166 Amino Acids)

Beta Interferon

- Contain 166 amino acids, only glycosylated.
- Two subtypes presents.
- Mainly produced by fibroblasts, epithelial cells and macrophages. Different types of interferon beta are used in human therapeutics: interferon beta-1a (produced in mammalian cells), and interferon beta-1b (produced in bacteria).
- It acts on type I receptor (although the mode of interaction with the receptor is different from that of interferon alpha, with interferon beta selectively induces phosphorylation of an alpha subunit-associated protein).
- Interferon beta is used to treat the relapsing-remitting form of **Multiple Sclerosis** (A disorder of the central nervous system [brain and spinal cord] involving decreased nerve function associated with the formation of scars on the covering of nerve cells).
- Betaseron -**Beta Interferon** from Berlex Laboratories, Inc.

Gamma Interferon

- Contain 146 amino acids, glycosylated
- Only one subtypes presents.
- Produced by T-lymphocytes (natural killer cells) only.

- It acts on type II receptor.
- Gamma interferon helps fight infections and tumors. Gamma interferon is used to treat chronic **granulomatous disease**. Trials are being conducted in India with gamma interferon as an anti TB drug.
- **Gammaron**–Interferon gamma from CIGB, Cuba.

Characteristics of the three main types of human interferon are discussed in the following table (112-117).

Table 3.1: Three Different Interferon

	Interferon Alpha (Type I)	*Interferon beta (Type I)*	*Interferon Gamma (Type II)*
Number of subtypes	At least 25	2	1
Structure	166 amino acids	166 amino acids, glycosylated	146 amino acids, glycosylated
Main origin	Mainly produced by leukocytes (white blood cells derived from bone marrow).	Mainly produced by fibroblasts, epithelial cells and macrophages. Different types of interferon beta are used in human therapeutics: interferon beta-1a (produced in mammalian cells), and interferon beta-1b (produced in bacteria).	Produced by T-lymphocytes (natural killer cells) only.
Receptor	Type I (multi-subunit receptor)	Type I (although the mode of interaction with the receptor is different from that of interferon alpha, with interferon beta selectively inducing phosphorylation of an alpha subunit-associated protein)	Type II

Biological Properties of Interferon

Interferon shows following biological response modifier-

1. Antiviral
2. Anti-proliferative
3. Immunomodulator activity.

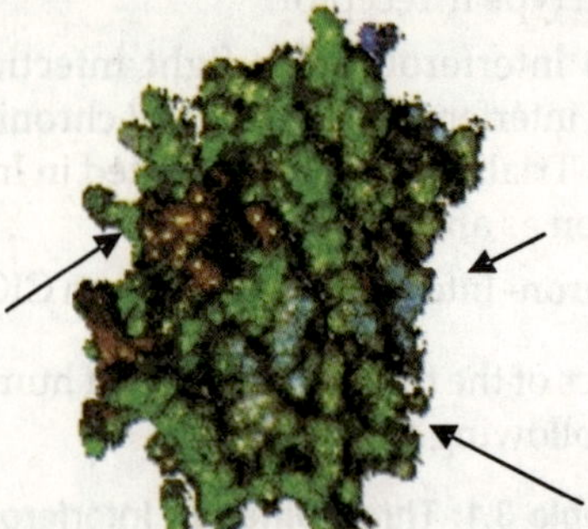

Fig. 3.3: Interferon Beta (Contain 166 Amino Acids, Only Glycosylated which are Pointed with Different Color Other than Green and Arrow).

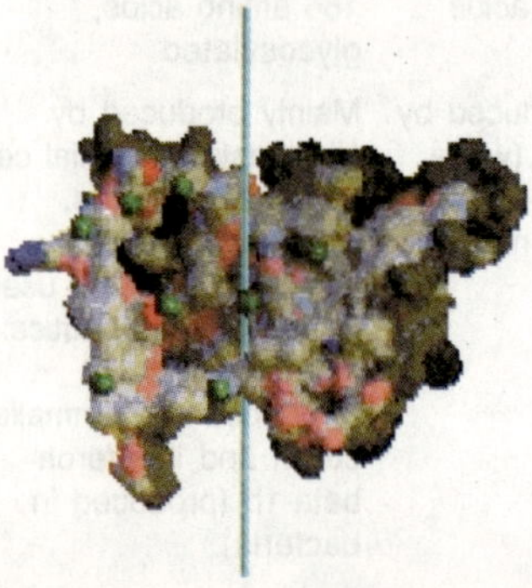

Fig. 3.4: Interferon Gamma (Contain 146 Amino Acids, Glycosylated)

Antiviral Effect

The antiviral effect of **Interferon** has been tested in several cell virus system showing all the properties for interferon alpha. Both DNA and RNA virus replication is inhibited.

In the case of retrovirus, the assembly of viral particles is inhibited. In papilloma virus infected cells **Interferon** has been shown to inhibit the expression of viral gene (26).

Antiproliferative Activity

Concerning the antiproliferative activity, interferon is the first natural protein observed with a negative regulatory action on growth, having an antigenic interactions with all known growth factors. **The effect is cytostatic rather than cytotoxic**, reversible and in transformed cells a morphological and functional regression towards non-transformed phenotype occurs after a prolonged treatment. The antiproliferative effect of **Interferon** has been equally characterized in several transformed cell lines, in vitro and in tumor xenograft bearing nude mouse (118, 119).

Immunomodulating Effect

The immunomodulating effect of interferon includes on various elements of the immune system such as stimulation of natural killer cells, specific cytotoxic T lymphocytes and macrophage tumor cell-lytic activities; modification of antibody production by B lymphocytes; regulation of HLA antigens expression on cell membranes and stimulation of interferon alpha production. These effects have been demonstrated for Interferon and play a relevant role in its therapeutically actions particularly anti-tumor (109-111).

Colony Stimulating Factors and Granulocyte Colony Stimulating Factor (GCSF), Granulocyte Macrophage Colony Stimulating Factor (GM-CSF)

Colony stimulating factors (CSF) are named according to the target cell type whose colony formation in soft agar cultures of bone marrow they induce. Of the CSF's, granulocyte-CSF (G-CSF) and granulocyte macrophage-CSF (GM-CSF) participate in acute inflammation. G-CSF was cloned in 1986 and its gene was mapped to chromosome 17 (112-117). It is a non-glycosylated protein of 19 kDa molecular weight. GM-CSF is a 22 kDa protein. Its full length cDNA sequence was obtained in 1985 and its gene was mapped to chromosome 5 in humans. Monocytes, T cells, fibroblasts and endothelial cells activated by macrophage products such as IL-1 or TNF, can produce G-CSF and GM-CSF. Both CSF's can stimulate neutrophils, while GM-CSF can also activate effector functions of eosinophils and mononuclear phagocytes. An example of the pathophysiologic role of GM-CSF is the airway inflammation accompanying asthma, where the implicated cytokines include IL-3, IL-5, and GM-CSF which perpetuate eosinophil activation and survival. In this scenario, the source of GM-CSF may be the alveolar macrophages which are reported to produce two to three fold higher levels of GM-CSF than control macrophages. Another possible source for all three cytokines are T cells present in the airways. Additional cytokines such IL-4, IL-13 (both stimulatory) and IFN-8 (inhibitory) may be involved in the control of IgE synthesis, while IL-1 and TNF-α may contribute to the airway inflammation by upregulation of endothelial adhesion molecule expression (78).

Granulocyte Colony Stimulating Factor (GCSF) is a protein stimulator of bone marrow cells, especially those of neutrophil lineage. Human GCSF is an 18.7 kDa protein containing 174 amino acid residues.

In addition, G-CSF can enhance the survival and activate the immunological functions mature neutrophils. (G-CSF) is a glycoprotein, which stimulates the survival, proliferation, differentiation and function of neutrophils, granulocytes, progenitor cells and mature neurtrophils (73).

Recombinant Human Granulocyte Colony Stimulating Factor (r Hu GCSF) application causes significantly reduction of patients primary and idiopathic neutropenia, aplastic anemia and also applicable in the indication malignant hematological diseases bone-marrow transplantation, peripheral blood stem cell transplantation, peripheral blood stem cell transplantation, mylodyplasia syndrome and patients who receive chemotherapy (75).

Insulin

The introduction of insulin was a breakthrough in the treatment of diabetes and it produced a remarkable increase in the life expectancy of diabetic patients. Animal-derived insulins have been used to treat people with diabetes since insulin was first discovered and continuously subjected to various purification technologies. Genetically engineered human insulin was introduced in 1982 and now the vast majority of people requiring insulin treatment worldwide are prescribed human insulin.

Insulin injections are needed in all patients with Type 1 (insulin dependent) diabetes right from the time of diagnosis of diabetes. In Type 2 (non-insulin dependent) diabetic patients, insulin is needed in those with primary or secondary failure to oral hypoglycemic agents and at times of stress like infection, myocardial infarction, etc. Insulin is also indicated in diabetes complicating pregnancy and gestational diabetes. The primary goal of treatment of diabetes is maintenance of near-normoglycemia to significantly reduce the risks for long-term microvascular complications of diabetes1.

Today physicians have the choice of at least 10 to 12 different insulin preparations which are in the Indian market. The newer insulins available today differ from older insulins in purity, homogenicity and price. While conventional insulin preparations, though recrystallized, are often heavily contaminated with other proteins, the new insulins were highly purified or monocomponent, which means that contamination with proinsulin is less than 1 part per million (ppm). Again while the old insulins are mostly mixtures of beef and pork insulins, the new insulins are purified monospecies insulins human structure. With the emergence of recombinant technology, biosynthetic human insulin has become the preferred choice of insulin for many physicians.

The human insulin can be produced in bacteria by recombinant DNA technology because of its two advantageous characteristics. First, the human insulin does not require the post-translational modification such as glycosylation (addition of sugar), so the recombinant insulin synthesized by a bacterium should be active. The second advantage concerns the size of the molecule. Insulin is a small protein comprising of two polypeptide chains (**A-chain** of 21 amino acids and **B-chain** of 30 amino acids) linked together by a **disulfide bonds** between the cysteine amino acids. Before becoming an active mature insulin, the insulin is produced from pancreatic cells as preproinsulin, which contain four segments; (1) an N-terminal signal sequence of 16 amino acids, (2) a B-chain of 30 amino acids, (3) a C-chain of 33 amino acids, and (4) an A-chain of 21 amino acids. During the post-translational modification, the N-terminal and the C-peptide are cleaved off, and the disulfide bonds are formed between the A-chain and the B-chain.

Tumor Necrosis Factor (TNF)

Tumor necrosis factors-(TNF) a and b are cytokines that bind to common receptors on the surface of target cells and exhibit several common biological activities. Human TNF-α and TNF-β are of 17 and 25 kDa, respectively. Their corresponding cDNAs were cloned in 1984, and the genes encoding the factors have been mapped to

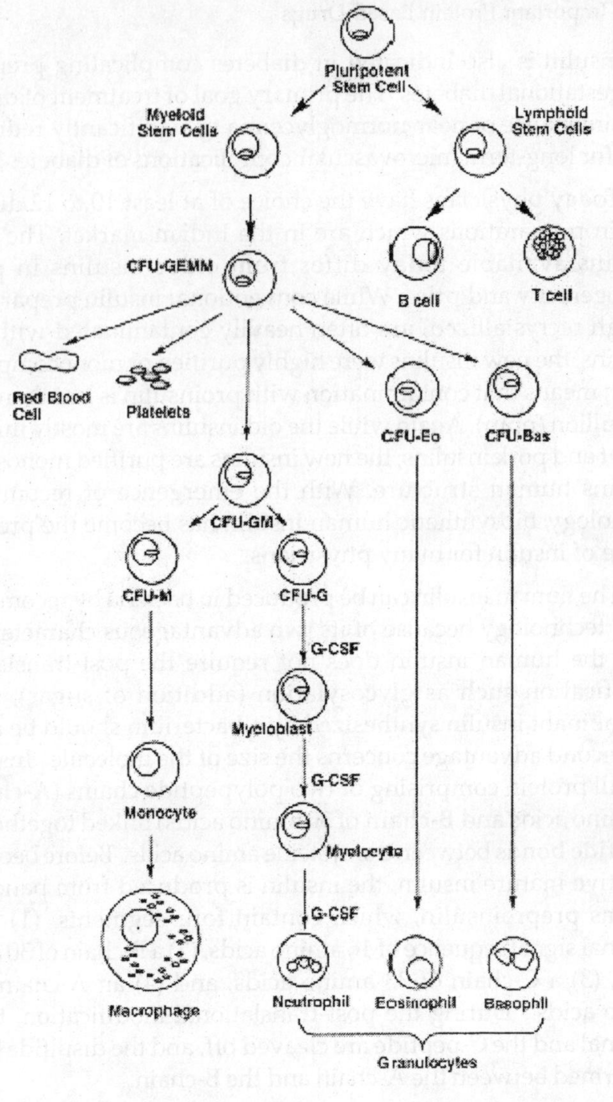

Fig. 3.5: Schematic Illustration of Hematopoiesis. The sites of action of G-CSF in this complex cascade are indicated (Ref 72, 73).

chromosome 6 in humans, within the region of the major histocompatibility complex (MHC). TNF-α, or cachectin, exists as a trimer and is one of the products of activated macrophages/ monocytes, fibroblasts, mast cells, and some T and natural killer (NK) cells.TNF-α and IL-1 share several pro-inflammatory properties. Like IL-1, TNF- α can induce fever, either directly via stimulation of PGE2 synthesis by the vascular endothelium of the hypothalamus, or indirectly by inducing release of IL-1. Both cytokines can stimulate the production of collagenase and PGE2 by synovial cells and thus are believed to contribute to joint damage in inflammatory conditions such as rheumatoid arthritis. TNF-α also shares an important inflammatory property with IL-6 and IL-11, *i.e.* the induction of acute phase reactant protein production by the liver. TNF-α and IL-1 further exert secondary inflammatory effects by stimulating IL-6 synthesis in several cell types. IL-6 then mediates its own effects and those of TNF-α and IL-1 in inducing fever and the acute phase response, thereby perpetuating the inflammatory response through a cascade of cytokines with overlapping properties. TNF-β, also known as lymphotoxin, is produced by activated T and B lymphocytes. It binds to the same high affinity receptors as TNF-α. Its properties are similar to those of TNF-α and include the induction of apoptosis (programmed cell death) in many types of transformed, virally infected, and tumor cells, and the stimulation of several PMN effector functions (39-42).

Although in general the effects of cytokines are exerted locally at the site of their production (autocrine and paracrine), TNF-α and TNF-β, as well as IL-1 and IL-6, have major systemic (endocrine) effects when either produced acutely in large amounts, as in the case of bacterial sepsis, or chronically in lesser amounts, as in the case of chronic infections. During sepsis with gram negative organisms, lipopolysaccharides (endotoxin) released from bacteria trigger the widespread production of TNF-α (and subsequently IL-1 and IL-6) by macrophages. The systemic release of these cytokines has been shown to be responsible for the fever and hypotension that characterize septic shock. In an analogous fashion, the production of large amounts of TNF-β by T lymphocytes in response to "superantigens" such as staphylococcal toxic shock syndrome toxin and enterotoxins are responsible for many of the systemic manifestations (fever, hypotension) of infections with toxin-producing gram positive organisms (128, 129). In addition, the

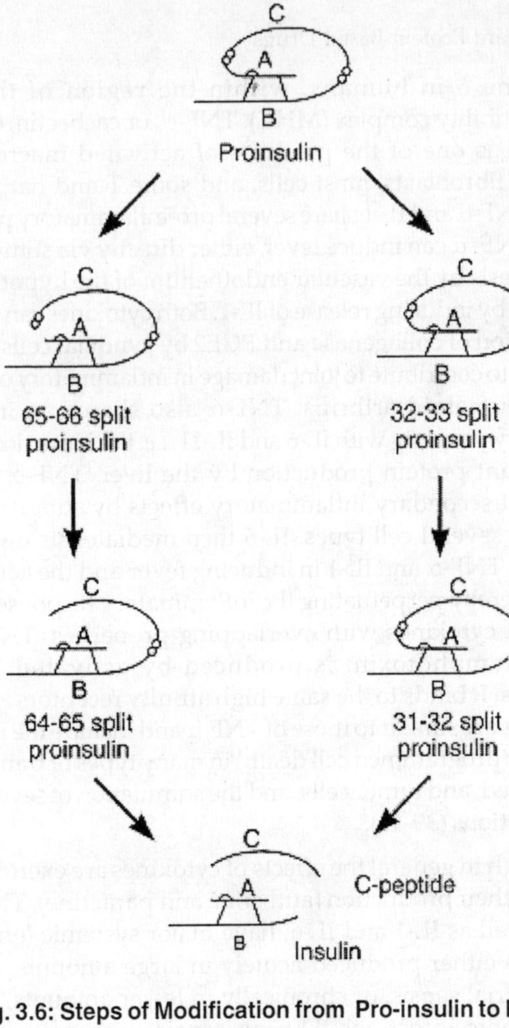

Fig. 3.6: Steps of Modification from Pro-insulin to Insulin.

chronic production of TNF is believed to be responsible for the metabolic alterations which result in the cachexia associated with chronic parasitic infections and some cancers (44, 45).

Interleukin-1

The cDNAs for IL-1α and β were cloned in 1984. They are encoded by two different genes, both located on human chromosome

2. Their size ranges from 22-31 kDa for cell-associated molecules, and 17.5 kDa for the secreted molecule. Their main cellular sources are mononuclear phagocytes, fibroblasts, keratinocytes, and T and B lymphocytes. Previous synonyms—endogenous pyrogen (EP), mononuclear cell factor, and lymphocyte-activating factor (LAF)—emphasize the role of IL-1 in inflammation. Both IL-1α and IL-1β can trigger fever by enhancing prostaglandin E2 (PGE2) synthesis by the vascular endothelium of the hypothalamus and can stimulate T cell proliferation. In addition, IL-1 elicits the release of histamine from mast cells at the site of inflammation. Histamine then triggers early vasodilation and increase of vascular permeability. The pro-inflammatory effects of IL-1 can be inhibited by IL-1 receptor antagonist (IL-1Ra), originally referred to as IL-1 inhibitor. IL-1Ra is produced by immune complex- or IL-4-stimulated macrophages and by TNF- or GM-CSF-stimulated neutrophils (100-102). It bears approximately 20-25% homology at the amino acid level to IL-1α and IL-1β. IL-1Ra inhibits IL-1 action by competing with IL-1 for binding to the IL-1 receptor (IL-1R) (40, 41).

Interleukin-2

The human IL-2 cDNA was cloned in 1983 and the corresponding gene has been mapped to the long arm of chromosome 4. IL-2 is a 15 kDa glycoprotein originally known as T cell growth factor (TCGF). It is secreted mainly by activated T helper cells. It acts as a growth factor/activator for T cells, NK cells, and B cells and promotes the development lymphokine-activated killer (LAK) cells (96). It therefore plays a critical role in regulating both cellular and humoral chronic inflammatory responses. Binding of IL-2 to the IL-2 receptor on T lymphocytes leads to cell proliferation, increased lymphokine secretion (IFN-γ, lymphotoxin, IL-4, IL-3, IL-5, GM-CSF), and enhanced expression class II MHC molecules (89, 121-123).

It is licensed for use by intravenous infusion in metastatic renal cell carcinoma (46-48).

Interleukin-6

Previous synonyms of IL-6 illustrate some its biologic activities. They include interferon-β (IFN-β2), hybridoma/plasmacytoma growth factor, hepatocyte-stimulating factor, B cell stimulatory factor 2 (BSF-2), and B cell differentiation factor BCDF). IL-6 is a glycoprotein ranging from 21 to 28 kDa depending on the degree of post-translational modification (124). The IL-6 cDNA was cloned in 1986 and the gene encoding IL-6 was mapped to chromosome 7 humans. IL-6 is produced by a variety of cells including mononuclear phagocytes, T cells, and fibroblasts. In addition to the stimulation of acute phase protein synthesis by the liver, IL-6 acts as growth factor for mature B cells and induces their final maturation into antibody-producing plasma cells. It is involved in T cell activation and differentiation, and participates in the induction of IL-β and IL-2 receptor expression (120). Some of the regulatory effects of IL-6 involve inhibition of TNF production, providing negative feedback for limiting the acute inflammatory response. Upregulation of IL-6 production has been observed in variety of chronic inflammatory and autoimmune disorders such as thyroiditis, type I diabetes, rheumatoid arthritis, systemic sclerosis, mesangial proliferative glomerulonephritis and psoriasis, and neoplasms such as cardiac myxoma, renal cell carcinoma, multiple myeloma, lymphoma, and leukemia (49-54).

Interleukin-8/Chemokines

IL-8 and other low molecular weight chemokines (*e.g.* platelet factor 4, IP-10, mig, ENA-78, macrophage inflammatory protein (MIP)-1a and b, MIP-2, monocyte chemoattractant protein-1 (MCP-1/JE), RANTES) belong to a chemotactic cytokine family and are responsible for the chemotactic migration and activation of neutrophils and other cell types (such as monocytes, lymphocytes, basophils, and eosinophils) at sites of inflammation. The two subsets of the chemokine family, "CXC" (or a), "C-C" (or b) are divided based on presence or absence of an amino acid between the first two of four conserved cysteines. A recent third subset, "C", has only two cysteines and to date only one member, IL-16, has been identified. Chemokines have been implicated in inflammatory conditions from acute neutrophil-mediated conditions such as acute respiratory distress syndrome to allergic asthma, arthritis, psoriasis, and chronic inflammatory disorders. To date, at least 27 chemokines have been described. The product of many cell types, including mononuclear phagocytes, antigen-activated T cells, endothelial and epithelial cells, and even neutrophils, IL-8 was previously known as neutrophil chemotactic factor (NCF) and neutrophil activating protein (NAP-1). It is the most thoroughly studied chemokine and therefore serves as a prototype for discussing the biologic properties of this rapidly

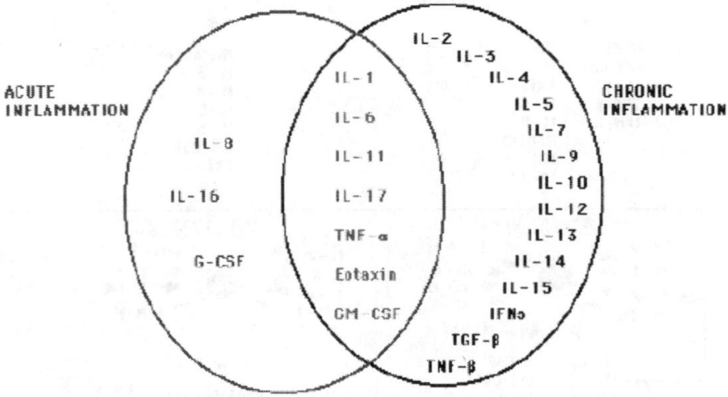

Fig. 3.7: Cytokines Involved in Acute and Chronic Inflammatory Responses (Ref. 55, 56).

growing family of inflammatory mediators. It consists of a 6-8 kDa protein whose cDNA was cloned by three different laboratories between 1987 and 1989 (60-64).

The corresponding gene has been mapped to chromosome 4 in humans. Its main inflammatory impact lies in its chemotactic effects on neutrophils and its ability to stimulate granulocyte activity. In addition, IL-8, IL-1, and TNF are involved in neutrophil recruitment by upregulating cell-surface adhesion molecule expression (such as endothelial leukocyte adhesion molecule, ELAM-1, and intracellular adhesion molecule, ICAM-1), thereby enhancing neutrophil adherence to endothelial cells 2) and facilitating their diapedesis through vessel walls. Thus, IL-8 mediates the recruitment and activation of neutrophils in inflamed tissue. IL-8 can be detected in synovial fluid from patients with various inflammatory rheumatic diseases, and mucosal levels of IL-8 are elevated in patients with active ulcerative colitis.Other members of this cytokine family, such as NAP-2, GROα, GROβ, GROγ, ENA-78, RANTES, MCP-1, MCP-2, MCP-3, platelet factor 4, MIP-1α/β, and MIP-2, are also likely to play important roles in acute inflammation via their shared effects on cell migration. MCP-1 is a chemokine identified in supernatants of blood mononuclear cells. Its production in monocytes is enhanced by inflammatory cytokines. MIP-1α and MIP-1β induce monocyte

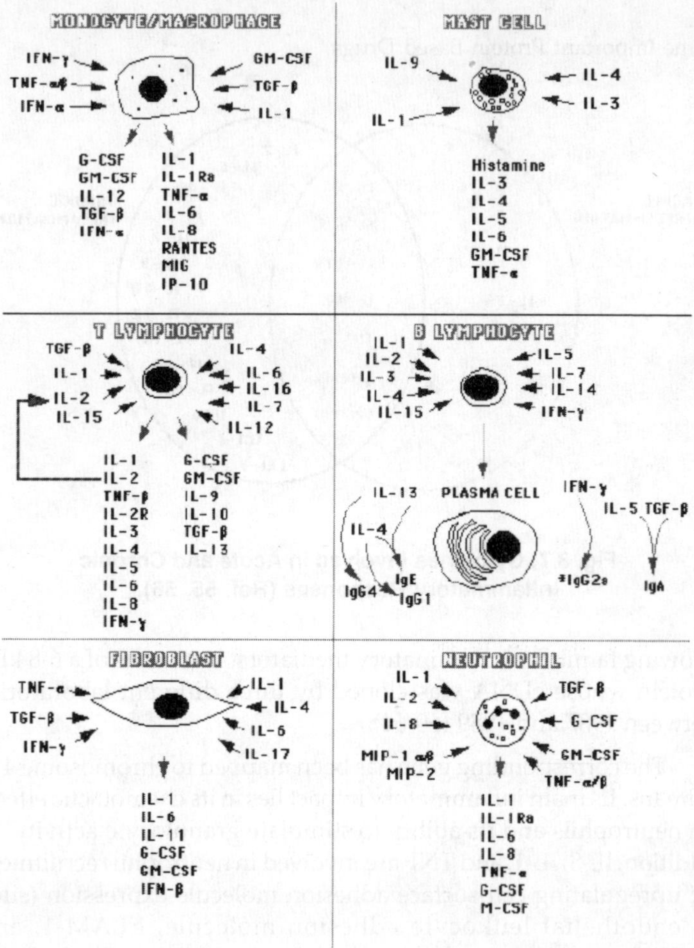

Fig. 3.8: Inflammatory Cytokines, Their Primary Sources and Target Cells (Ref. 40, 113, 125-127).

and T lymphocyte migration. MIP-1a , MCP-1, and MIP-2 have been implicated in the pathogenesis of rheumatoid arthritis where they are believed to recruit mononuclear cells into the inflamed regions of the synovium. Several other members of the IL-8/chemokine family have been identified but their biologic effects are as yet poorly defined.

Two recently identified chemokines, eotaxin and IL-16, have some unique properties and are described below (85-88).

Interleukin-16

IL-16 was originally identified as a chemotactic factor known as lymphocyte chemoattractant factor or lymphotactin. It is the only member of the "C" family of chemokines. The gene encoding IL-16 has been mapped to human chromosome 1. IL-16 is an unusual cytokine in that preformed IL-16 is stored in CD8+ lymphocytes and is secreted upon stimulation with histamine or serotonin. It induces chemotaxis of CD4+ T lymphocytes and is believed to initiate T-cell mediated inflammation in asthma (67).

Interleukin-17

The human IL-17 cDNA was cloned in 1995 based on homology with murine CTLA8. A 1.9 Kb cDNA was found to encode a protein of 17.5 kDa homologous to a product of Herpesvirus saimiri (HVS13). IL-17 is a product of activated T lymphocytes and its biologic activities include stimulation of IL-6 and IL-8 production and enhanced ICAM-1 expression on human foreskin fibroblasts (57-59).

Interleukin-3

IL-3, also called multi-CSF, is produced by activated T cells and mast cells. The molecular weight of IL-3 ranges from 14 to 36 kDa. The cloning of the corresponding cDNA was reported in 1984, and the IL-3 gene has been localized to chromosome 5. It stimulates eosinophils and B cell differentiation while it inhibits lymphokine-activated killer (LAK) cell activity. IL-3 shares several biological activities with GM-CSF (76).

Interleukin-4

IL-4 is expressed as a 15-19 kDa protein and exists as a dimer. The IL-4 gene has been mapped to human chromosome 5, and the corresponding cDNA was cloned in 1986. IL-4 is produced by CD4+ (TH) cells, mast cells, and basophils. It induces CD4+ T cells to differentiate into TH2 cells while suppressing the development of TH1 cells (80). It also acts as a B cell, T cell, and mast cell growth factor, it enhances class II MHC expression on B cells, and it promotes immunoglobulin class switching to IgG1 and IgE. In fact, IL-4 is necessary for IgE response induction, and its absence also leads to significantly lower levels of IgG1 in T cell-dependent immune responses. The stimulatory effects of IL-4 on IgG1 and IgE production and on MHC class II induction are downregulated by IFN-γ, a cytokine whose functions are antagonized by IL-4 and vice versa. IL-4 also stimulates collagen and IL-6 production by human dermal fibroblasts, and may thus play a role in the pathogenesis of fibrotic diseases such as systemic sclerosis. In rheumatoid arthritis, on the other hand, IL-4 appears to exhibit some anti-inflammatory properties by inhibiting the production of several proinflammatory cytokines such as IL-1, IL-6, IL-8, and TNF-α, by synovial membranes of rheumatoid arthritis patients (79, 81-84).

Interleukin-5

Cloned in 1987, the IL-5 cDNA encodes a protein of 20-22 kDa which has an apparent molecular weight of 45 kDa upon dimerization. Like IL-4, the gene for IL-5 has also been mapped to chromosome 5 in humans. IL-5, also known as B cell growth factor II (BCGFII) and T cell replacing factor (TRF), is produced by CD4+ T helper cells as well as NK cells, and exists as a dimer linked by disulfide bonds. IL-5 is involved in eosinophil differentiation and activation and stimulation of immunoglobulin class switching to IgA. Other properties of IL-5 include increased activation of B cell proliferation, and enhancement of T cell cytotoxicity. The combined production of IL-4 and IL-5 by CD4+ TH2 cells therefore results in IgE and IgA production and mast cell and eosinophil stimulation (65, 66).

Interleukin-7

IL-7 is a cytokine of about 25 kDa whose cDNA was cloned in 1989. Its gene has been mapped to human chromosome 8. IL-7, a cytokine purified as a pre-B cell growth factor, is a bone marrow and thymic stromal cell product. It stimulates the development of pre-B and pre-T cells and acts as a growth factor for B cells, T cells, and early thymocytes.

Interleukin-9

IL-9 is another cytokine produced by CD4+ T helper (TH2) cells as well as some B lymphomas. First described in the mouse, IL-9 was known as mast cell growth-enhancing activity (MEA) and murine Tcell growth factor P40. The IL-9 cDNA was cloned in 1989 and the gene encoding it was mapped to human chromosome 5. Its production is IL-4 and IL-10, and thus IL-2-dependent. IL-9 is regulatory in nature in that it inhibits lymphokine production by IFN-γ-producing CD4+ T cells and enhances the growth of CD8+ T cells. In addition, IL-9 promotes the production of immunoglobulins by B cells and the proliferation of mast cells.

Interleukin-10

IL-10 is also referred to as B cell-derived T cell growth factor and cytokine synthesis inhibitory factor (CSIF) because it inhibits IFN-γ production by activated T cells. The cDNA for human IL-10 was cloned in 1990 and found to encode an 18 kDa protein. IL-10 is produced by a variety of cell types, including CD4+ T cells, activated CD8+ T cells, and activated B cells. Its effects include reduction of antigen-specific T cell proliferation, inhibition of IL- 2-induced IFN-γ production by NK cells, and inhibition of IL-4 and IFN-γ induced MHC class II expression on monocytes. Since IL-10 can be produced by TH2 cells and inhibits TH1 function by preventing TH1 cytokine production (such as IFN-γ), IL-10 is considered a T cell cross-regulatory factor and has thus been referred to as an "anticytokine". IL-10 also acts as a co-differentiation factor for cytotoxic T cells and a co-factor for T cell growth (69-74). Human IL-10 (hIL-10) shares 84% identity at the amino acid level with a homolog, viral IL-10 (vIL-10), which is encoded by the Epstein-Barr virus. vIL-10 shares with hIL-10 inhibitory effects on cytokine production and stimulatory effects on B cell growth (91-95).

Interleukin-13

IL-13 was originally identified as a protein produced by activated murine TH2 lymphocytes and referred to as P600. The cDNA for IL-13 was recently cloned and the gene was mapped to human chromosome 5, closely linked to the gene encoding IL-4. A 12-17 kDa protein, IL-13 exhibits anti-inflammatory activities by inhibiting the production of inflammatory cytokines, such as IL-1b, TNF-α, IL-8, and IL-6, by human peripheral blood monocytes induced with lipopolysaccharide. Inhibition of inflammatory cytokine production is also a characteristic of two other cytokines produced by TH2 lymphocytes, namely IL-4 and IL-10. In addition, IL-13 enhances monocyte and B lymphocyte differentiation and proliferation, increases CD23 expression, and induces IgG4 and IgE class switching (97, 98).

Interleukin-14

A product of malignant B and T cells as well as normal T cells, IL-14 is a 53 kDa B-cell growth factor (BCGF). Like IL-4, IL-14 has been shown to induce B cell proliferation. However, IL-14 inhibits immunoglobulin secretion. It has been suggested to play an important role in the aggressive form of B-cell type non-Hodgkin's lymphoma (99).

Interleukin-12

IL-12, previously known as natural killer cell stimulatory factor (NKSF) and cytotoxic lymphocyte maturation factor (CLMF), was originally isolated from Epstein-Barr virus transformed B cells. It is a heterodimer composed of two subunits of 35 and 40 kDa. The cDNAs for both subunits were cloned in 1991. Its biological activities include enhancement of cytotoxic T cells and lymphokineactivated killer (LAK) cell generation and activation, increased natural killer (NK) cell cytotoxicity, induction of activated T cell and NK cell proliferation, induction of IFN-γ production by NK cells and T cells, and inhibition of IgE synthesis by IL-4-stimulated lymphocytes via IFN-γ-dependent and independent mechanisms. IL-12 is secreted by activated B cells, macrophages, and other antigen-presenting cells (APCs), but its production is inhibited by IL-4 and IL-10. In addition, the stimulatory effect of IL-12 on TH1 development is antagonized by IL-4, a cytokine which promotes TH2 cell development. Therefore, IL-12 plays an important role in cell-mediated inflammation and also contributes to the regulation of immunoglobulin production (103-105).

Interleukin-15

IL-15 is a cytokine of approximately 15 kDa originally discovered as a T cell stimulatory activity produced by activated monocytes, epithelial cells, and fibroblasts. IL-15 shares many biologic properties with IL-2 and mediates its activity via a multi-subunit high affinity receptor comprised of a unique alpha chain and the beta and gamma chains of the IL-2R. The human IL-15 gene has been mapped to chromosome 4, similarly to IL-2. However, IL-15 does not exhibit any sequence homology with IL-2. IL-15 is produced by a large variety of cells including T lymphocytes and monocytes. It stimulates T lymphocyte and NK cell proliferation, as well as CTL and LAK activity. It enhances B cell expansion and immunoglobulin production. It is also a T lymphocyte chemoattractant. IL-15 may be responsible for the recruitment and activation of T lymphocytes in the synovium of patients with rheumatoid arthritis where its levels have been found to be elevated (106-108).

Some other important therapeutic proteins are :

Erythropoietin (EPO)

1. Kidney **glyco**protein that stimulates growth of red blood cells in bone marrow (note that the source of a glycoprotein is important.
2. Approx. equal mass of protein (34 kD) and carbohydrate
3. Used in anemia

Blood Factor: Factor VIII

Involved in cascade associated with blood clotting Factor VIII is missing in hemophilia A, Factor VIII from blood products used to treat hemophilia; this led to some of the earliest cases of AIDS transmission from human blood (130-133).

Emphasizes the importance of avoiding human based products.

Deficiency of the factor VIII protein results in the X-linked recessive disorder of haemophilia A. The principle clinical features of haemophilia A are bleeding into the joints, which are often swollen and painful, this can result in impaired mobility and degenerative arthritis. Bleeding in to muscles can cause necrosis, contractures and neuropathy. Prolonged bleeding from cuts and frequent bruising are common. Clinically the disorder is very heterogeneous. Patients are generally classed as severely, moderately or mildly affected, the clinical severity correlates with coagulation factor VIII activities that are <2%, 2-5%, and 5-30% of normal levels. In the UK about 40% of haemophilia A patients are classed as severely affected. Treatment is by replacement therapy using factor VIII derived from human plasma or recombinant factor VIII.

Blood Factor: Factor IX

The molecular weight of human Factor IX protein ranges from 55,000 to 71,000 Daltons (55-71 kDa).

Factor IX is a protein produced naturally in the body. It helps the blood form clots to stop bleeding. Injections of factor IX are used to treat hemophilia B, which is sometimes called Christmas disease. This is a condition in which the body does not make enough factor IX. If you do not have enough factor IX and you become injured, your blood will not form clots as it should, and you may bleed into and damage your muscles and joints.

Injections of one form of factor IX, called factor IX complex, also are used to treat certain people with hemophilia A. In hemophilia A, sometimes called classical hemophilia, the body does not make enough factor VIII, and, just as in hemophilia B, the blood cannot form clots as it should. Injections of factor IX complex may be used in patients in whom the medicine used to treat hemophilia A is no longer effective. The factor IX product is obtained naturally from human blood or artificially by a man-made process. Factor IX obtained from human blood has been treated and is not likely to contain harmful viruses such as hepatitis B virus, hepatitis C (non-A, non-B) virus, or human immunodeficiency virus (HIV), the virus that causes acquired immunodeficiency syndrome (AIDS). The man-made factor IX product does not contain these viruses (68, 130-133).

Growth Factors

Proteins involved in controlling differentiation and production of various cell types:

EGF

Epidermal growth factor, wound healing

IGF

Insulin-like growth factor, promotes tissue growth, nutritional and growth disorders

PDGF

Platelet-derived growth factors, collagen deposition in tissue repair Becaplermin (topical gel formulation): treatment of diabetic ulcers of the lower extremities

Epidermal Growth Factor (EGF)

Studies based on observation that some animals lick their wounds resulted in isolation of a factor name EGF-Epidermal Growth Factor, obtained from sub-maxilary and Sublingual glands of Mice. EGF was also obtained from human urine.

EGF is 53 amino acid peptide chain. It is a ubiquitous molecule like other growth factors and contrary to the classic hormones.

EGF stimulates in vitro proliferation of both fibroblasts and epithelial cells. Evidence have been collected the healing properties of EGF in experimental models.

There are reports of EGF is capable of accelerating the healing of skin burn on hog contributing to a better physiological regeneration of damaged epithelium thus offering functional and aesthetic advantages.

It was reported that EGF provokes a faster growth of cellular colonies in skin culture. And also reported that the effected of EGF on the sub-epithelial portion of a wound stimulated early fibroblasts with a linear orientation while the control wounds had a greater disorganization. Cases treated with EGF showed a more orderly visualization. Understanding connective tissue matured faster while the contraction of the wound was notably shower in the control group.

It was reported an EGF provoked mitogeneric effect on fibroblasts and ephithelial cells. Furthermore, EGF is capable of stimulating all other cellular elements of a wound. The healing of wounds treated with EGF resembles the normal surrounding tissue, with less deformity when compared to the control group (87).

It was demonstrated that topical applications of EGF on experimental animals accelerated epidermal accelerated epidermal regeneration in case of burns diabetic ulcers and skin graft donation areas.

Vascular Endothelial Growth Factor

Angiogenesis is a process of new blood vessel development from pre-existing vasculature. It plays an essential role in embryonic development, nor mal growth of tissues, wound healing, the female reproductive cycle (*i.e.,* ovulation, menstruation and placental development), as well as a major role in many diseases. Particular interest has focused on cancer, since tumors cannot grow be yond a few millimeters in size with out developing a new blood supply. Angiogenesis is also necessary for the spread and growth of tumor cell metastases One of the most important growth and survival factors for endothelium is vascular endothelial growth factor VEGF. VEGF induces angiogenesis and endothelial cell proliferation and it plays an important role in regulating vasculogenesis. VEGF is a heparin-binding glycoprotein that is secreted as a homodimer of 45 kDa. Most types of cells, but usually not endothelial cells them selves, secrete VEGF. Since the initially discovered VEGF, VEGF-A, in creases vascular permeability, it was known as vascular permeability factor. In addition, VEGF causes vasodilatation, partly through stimulation of nitric oxide synthasein endothelial cells. VEGF can also stimulate cell migration and inhibit apoptosis.

There are several splice variants of VEGF-A. The major ones in clude: 121, 165, 189 and 206 amino acids (aa), each one comprising a specific exon addition. VEGF165 is the most predominant protein, but transcripts of VEGF121 may be more abundant. VEGF206 is rarely ex pressed and has been detected only in fetal liver. Recently, other splice variants of 145 and 183 aa have also been de scribed. The 165, 189 and 206 aa splice variants have heparin-binding do mains, which help anchor them in extra cellular matrix and are involved in binding to heparin sulfate and presentation to VEGF receptors. This is a key factor for VEGF potency (*i.e.,* the heparin-binding forms are more active). Several other members of the VEGF family have been cloned including VEGF-B, -C, and -D. Placenta growth factor (PlGF) is also closely related to VEGF-A. VEGF-A, -B, -C, -D, and PlGF are all distantly related to platelet-derived growth factors-A and -B. Less is known about the function and regulation of VEGF-B, -C, and -D, but they do not seem to be regulated by the major path ways that regulate VEGF-A.

Human Growth Hormone (HGH, Somatotropin)

1. From pituitary gland, used for growth deficiencies in children (dwarfism).
2. Hormone isolated from human cadaver pituitary contained protein-associated infectious particles that co-purified with the hormone: lead to a viral like condition in some patients, (Jacob-Kreutzfeld syndrome) that leads to mental deterioration and death.
3. Only small amounts previously available, therefore, only limited amounts available for research into healing etc. due to ethical requirements.
4. Some more informations are as follows:

(a) 29 amino acid peptide that corresponds to the N-terminus of the 44 residue growth-hormone-releasing factor (GHRF).

(b) Stimulates release of HGH (most patients with HGH deficiency have adequate stores of the hormone in their pituitary).

(c) Lower cost that HGH but efficacy may be lower

Tissue Type Plasminogen Activator (tPA)

Tissue-type plasminogen activator (tPA) plays a key role in thrombus dissolution and plasma levels of tPA have been associated with cardiovascular disease.

tPA acts as a fibrinolytic drug by activating plasminogen to form plasmin, which degrades fibrin and breaks up thrombi. It is therefore indicated for use in dissolving the coronary artery blood clots associated with acute myocardial infarctions.

Streptokinase (STK)

Thrombolytic agents are used to dissolve blood clots that have formed in certain blood vessels. These medicines are usually used when a blood clot seriously lessens the flow of blood to certain parts of the body. Streptokinase (STK), a protein of 415 amino acids that does not contain disulfide bridges, is produced and excreted by some strains of ß-hemolytic streptococci. Because of its ability to activate the fibrinolytic system, it is currently used as a thrombolytic agent for the treatment of patients with acute myocardial infarction. The production of STK by methods yielding a high benefit/cost or benefit/risk ratio is highly desirable. One of those methods is recombinant.DNA technology that could be used to produce high quantities of recombinant STK that Avoiding the contamination risks that arise from the manipulation of pathogens such as those belonging to the streptococcus species.

Pharmacodynamics of Streptokinase (Biological Actions)

The blood fibrinolytic system involves the activation of blood plasminogen by various factors to form the enzyme plasmin. This is the stage at which streptokinase works. Plasmin is a proteolytic enzyme which degrades fibrin and hence dissolves the thrombus.

Streptokinase is not an enzyme but when it binds to plasminogen it forms an activator complex by which plasmin is formed. Normally there are naturally occurring inhibitors of plasmin (antiplasmins) in blood which prevent plasmin itself from being used as a fibrinolytic agent, whereas there are no such inhibitors for streptokinase. Plasmin formed inside a thrombus by streptokinase is protected from blood antiplasmins thus allowing it to dissolve the thrombus from within.

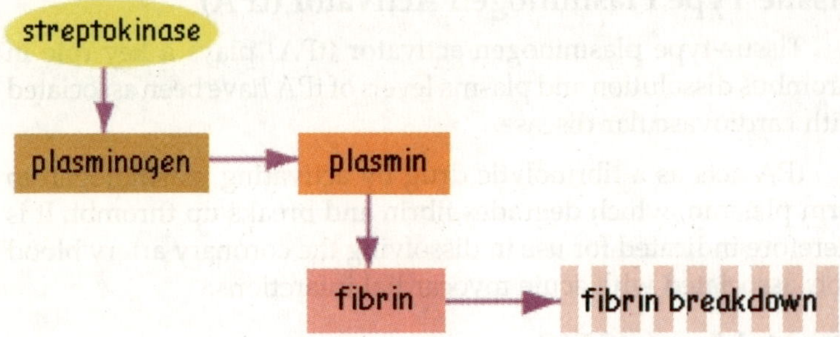

Fig. 3.9: Biological action of Streptokinase

Thyroid-Stimulating Hormone (Thyrotropin)

Thyroid-stimulating hormone, also known as thyrotropin, is secreted from cells in the anterior pituitary called *thyrotrophs*, finds its receptors on epithelial cells in the thyroid gland, and stimulates that gland to synthesize and release thyroid hormone.

TSH is a glycoprotein hormone composed of two subunits which are non-covalently bound to one another. The alpha subunit of TSH is also present in two other pituitary glycoprotein hormones, follicle-stimulating hormone and luteinizing hormone, and, in primates, in the placental hormone chorionic gonadotropin. Each of these hormones also has a unique beta subunit, which provides receptor specificity. In other words, TSH is composed of alpha subunit bound to the TSH beta subunit, and TSH associates only with its own receptor. Free alpha and beta subunits have essentially no biological activity.

The most important controller of TSH secretion is thyroid-releasing hormone. Thyroid-releasing hormone is secreted by hypothalamic neurons into hypothalamic-hypophyseal portal blood, finds its receptors on thyrotrophs in the anterior pituitary and stimulates secretion of TSH.

One interesting aspect of thyroid-releasing hormone is that it is only three amino acids long. Its basic sequence is glutamic acid-histidine-proline, although both ends of the peptide are modified.

Secretion of thyroid-releasing hormone, and hence, TSH, is inhibited by high blood levels of thyroid hormones in a classical negative feedback loop.

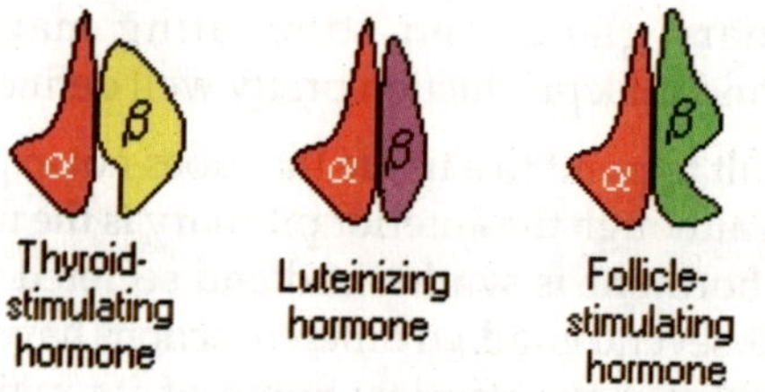

Fig. 3.10: Three important hormone – TSH, LH and FSH

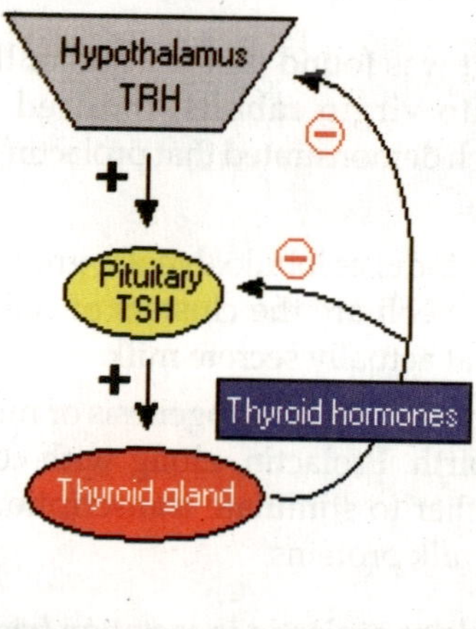

Fig. 3.11: Biological role and pathway Thyroid hormone

Prolactin

Prolactin is a single-chain protein hormone closely related to growth hormone. It is secreted by so-called *lactotrophs* in the anterior pituitary. It is also synthesized and secreted by a broad range of other cells in the body, most prominently various immune cells, the brain and the decidua of the pregnant uterus.

Prolactin is synthesized as a prohormone. Following cleavage of the signal peptide, the length of the mature hormone is between 194 and 199 amino acids, depending on species. Hormone structure is stabilized by three intramolecular disulfide bonds.

Physiologic Effects of Prolactin

The conventional view of prolactin is that its major target organ is the mammary gland, and stimulating mammary gland development and milk production pretty well define its functions.

It is difficult to point to a tissue that does not express prolactin receptors, and although the anterior pituitary is the major source of prolactin, the hormone is synthesized and secreted in many other tissues. Overall, several hundred different actions have been reported for prolactin in various species. Some of its major effects are summarized here.

Mammary Gland Development, Milk Production and Reproduction

In the 1920's it was found that extracts of the pituitary gland, when injected into virgin rabbits, induced milk production. Subsequent research demonstrated that prolactin has two major roles in milk production:

- Prolactin induces lobuloalveolar growth of the mammary gland. Alveoli are the clusters of cells in the mammary gland that actually secrete milk.
- Prolactin stimulates lactogenesis or milk production after giving birth. Prolactin, along with cortisol and insulin, act together to stimulate transcription of the genes that encode milk proteins

The critical role of prolactin in lactation has been confirmed in mice with targeted deletions in the prolactin gene. Female mice that are heterozygous for the deleted prolactin gene (and produce roughly half the normal amount of prolactin) show failure to lactate after their first pregnancy.

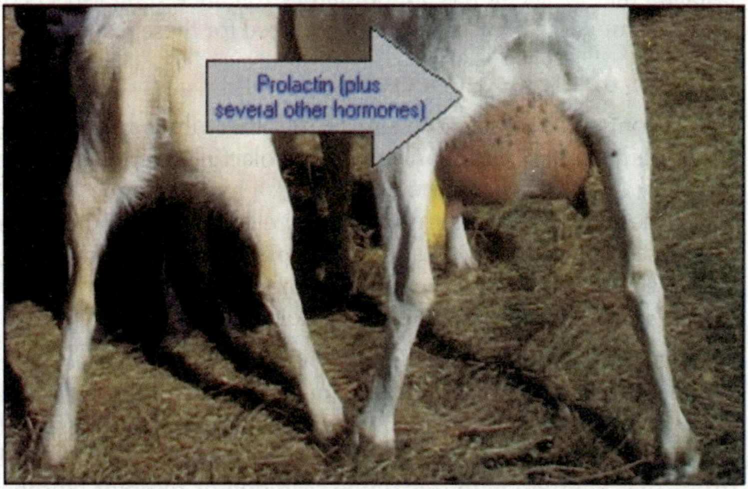

Fig. 3.12: Action of Prolactin (before use and after use)

Prolactin also appears important in several non-lactational aspects of reproduction. In some species (rodents, dogs, skunks), prolactin is necessary for maintainance of corpora lutea (ovarian structures that secrete progesterone, the "hormone of pregnancy"). Mice that are homozygous for an inactivated prolactin gene and thus incapable of secreting prolactin are infertile due to defects in ovulation, fertilization, preimplantation development and implantation.

Finally, prolactin appears to have stimulatory effects in some species on reproductive or maternal behaviors such as nest building and retrieval of scattered young.

Effects on Immune Function

The prolactin receptor is widely expressed by immune cells, and some types of lymphocytes synthesize and secrete prolactin. These observations suggest that prolactin may act as an autocrine or paracrine modulator of immune activity. Interestingly, mice with homozygous deletions of the prolactin gene fail to show significant abnormalities in immune responses.

A considerable amount of research is in progress to delineate the role of prolactin in normal and pathologic immune responses. It appears that prolactin has a modulatory role in several aspects of immune function, but is not strictly required for these responses.

Control of Prolactin Secretion

In contrast to what is seen with all the other pituitary hormones, the hypothalamus tonically suppresses prolactin secretion from the pituitary. In other words, there is usually a hypothalamic "brake" set on the lactotroph, and prolactin is secreted only when the brake is released. If the pituitary stalk is cut, prolactin secretion increases, while secretion of all the other pituitary hormones fall dramatically due to loss of hypothalamic releasing hormones.

Dopamine serves as the major prolactin-inhibiting factor or brake on prolactin secretion. Dopamine is secreted into portal blood by hypothalamic neurons, binds to receptors on lactotrophs, and inhibits both the synthesis and secretion of prolactin. Agents and drugs that interfere with dopamine secretion or receptor binding lead to enhanced secretion of prolactin.

In addition to tonic inhibition by dopamine, prolactin secretion is positively regulated by several hormones, including thyroid-releasing hormone, gonadotropin-releasing hormone and vasoactive intestinal polypeptide. Stimulation of the nipples and mammary gland, as occurs during nursing, leads to prolactin release. This effect appears to be due to a spinal reflex arc that causes release of prolactin-stimulating hormones from the hypothalamus.

Estrogens provide a well-studied positive control over prolactin synthesis and secretion. The increasing blood concentrations of estrogen during late pregnancy appear responsible for the elevated levels of prolactin that are necessary to prepare the mammary gland for lactation at the end of gestation.

Disease States

Excessive secretion of prolactin–hyperprolactinemia–is a relative common disorder in humans. This condition has numerous causes, including prolactin-secreting tumors and therapy with certain drugs.

Common manifestations of hyperprolactinemia in women include amenorrhea (lack of menstrural cycles) and galactorrhea (excessive or spontaneous secretion of milk). Men with hyperprolactinemia typically show hypogonadism, with decreased sex drive, decreased sperm production and impotence. Such men also often show breast enlargement (gynecomastia), but very rarely produce milk.

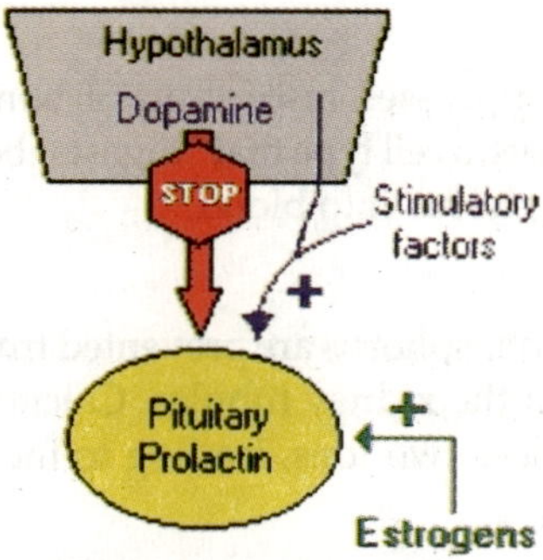

Fig. 3.13: Biological role and pathway of Prolactin

Calcitonin

Calcitonin is a hormone known to participate in calcium and phosphorus metabolism. In mammals, the major source of calcitonin is from the parafollicular or C cells in the thyroid gland, but it is also synthesized in a wide variety of other tissues, including the lung and intestinal tract. In birds, fish and amphibians, calcitonin is secreted from the ultimobrachial glands.

Calcitonin is a 32 amino acid peptide cleaved from a larger prohormone. It contains a single disulfide bond, which causes the amino terminus to assume the shape of a ring. Alternative splicing of the calcitonin pre-mRNA can yield a mRNA encoding calcitonin gene-related peptide; that peptide appears to function in the nervous and vascular systems. The calcitonin receptor has been cloned and shown to be a member of the seven-transmembrane, G protein-coupled receptor family.

Physiologic Effects of Calcitonin

A large and diverse set of effects has been attributed to calcitonin, but in many cases, these were seen in response to pharmacologic doses of the hormone, and their physiologic relevance is suspect. It seems clear however, that calcitonin plays a role in calcium and phosphorus metabolism. In particular, calcitonin has the ability to decrease blood calcium levels at least in part by effects on two well-studied target organs:

Bone

Calcitonin suppresses resorption of bone by inhibiting the activity of osteoclasts, a cell type that "digests" bone matrix, releasing calcium and phosphorus into blood.

Kidney

Calcium and phosphorus are prevented from being lost in urine by reabsorption in the kidney tubules. Calcitonin inhibits tubular reabsorption of these two ions, leading to increased rates of their loss in urine.

It seems clear that there are species differences in the importance of calcitonin as a factor affecting calcium homeostasis. In fish, rodents and some domestic animals, calcitonin appears to play a significant role in calcium homeostais. In humans, calcitonin has at best a minor role in regulating blood concentrations of calcium. One interesting piece of evidence to support this statement is that humans with chronically increased (medullary thyroid cancer) or decreased (surgical removal of the thyroid gland) levels of calcitonin in blood do not show alterations from normal in serum calcium concentration.

Control of Calcitonin Secretion

The most prominent factor controlling calcitonin secretion is the extracellular concentration of ionized calcium. Elevated blood calcium levels strongly stimulate calcitonin secretion, and secretion is suppressed when calcium concentration falls below normal. A number of other hormones have been shown to stimulate calcitonin release in certain situations, and nervous controls also have been demonstrated.

Disease States

A large number of diseases are associated with abnormally increased or decreased levels of calcitonin, but pathologic effects of abnormal calcitonin secretion *per se* are not generally recognized.

There are several therapeutic uses for calcitonin. It is used to treat hypercalcemia resulting from a number of causes, and has been a valuable therapy for Paget disease, which is a disorder in bone remodeling. Calcitonin also appears to be a valuable aid in the management of certain types of osteoporosis.

Insulin-like Growth Factor

Insulin-like growth factor is a basic peptide believed to be secreted by the liver and to circulate in the blood. Molecular weight of the protein 7.7 kD. It has growth-regulating, insulin-like, and mitogenic activities. This growth factor has a major, but not absolute, dependence on somatotropin. IGF-I is mainly active in adults in contrast to IGF-II, which is a major fetal growth factor.

Chapter 4

Production Process: Steps Involved

Development of Clones

In the early 1970s, biochemists at Stanford University showed that genetic traits could indeed be transferred from one organism to another. In this experiment, the DNA of one microorganism recombined with the inserted DNA sequence of another, and thus had been edited to exhibit a very specific modification.

The actual editing, or insertion process, is painstaking, for it involves manipulating incredibly tiny pieces of incredibly tiny organisms. But the process can be explained in terms of editing a written text: scissors and "glue" are used to "cut" and "paste."

The methods used in rDNA technology are fairly simple. We take, for example, the sentence (gene) for insulin production in humans and paste it into the DNA of *Escherichia coli*, a bacterium that inhabits the human digestive tract. The bacterial cells divide very rapidly making billions of copies of themselves, and each bacterium carries in its DNA a faithful replica of the gene for insulin production. Each new *E. coli* cell has inherited the human insulin gene sentence.

How do we transfer the gene embodying the instruction for therapeutic protein production? One approach would be to cut the appropriate gene from human DNA and paste, or splice, it into

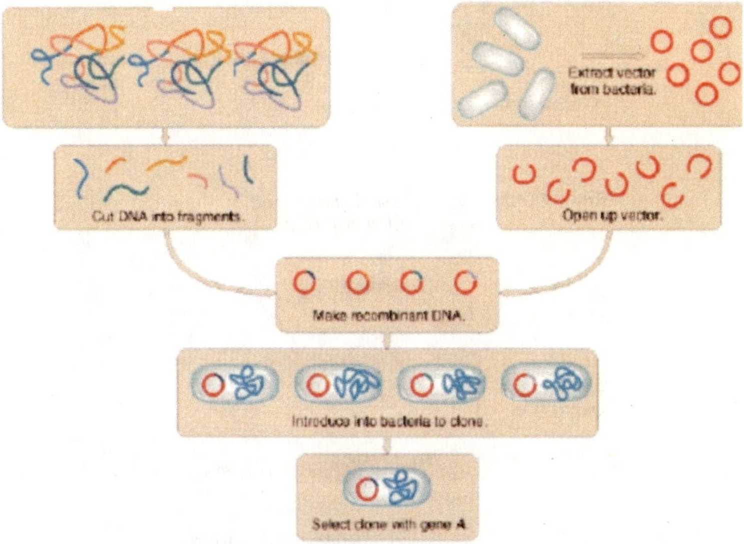

Fig. 4.1(A)

plasmid DNA, a special kind of DNA that takes a circular form and can be used as a vehicle for this editing job. Our "scissors" are the class of enzymes called restriction enzymes. There are well over a hundred restriction enzymes, each cutting in a very precise way a specific base sequence of the DNA molecule. With these scissors used singly or in various combinations, the segment of the human DNA molecule that specifies insulin production can be isolated (25).

This segment is "glued" into place using an enzyme called DNA ligase. The result is an edited, or recombinant, DNA molecule. When this recombinant plasmid DNA is inserted into E. coli, the cell will be able to process the instructions to assemble the amino acids for insulin production. More importantly, the new instructions are passed along to the next generation of *E. coli* cells in the process known as gene cloning.

Production in Fermentation

Bioreactors or fermentar are vessels in which raw materials are biologically converted into specific products, using MOs, plant, animal or human cells or individual enzymes. A bioreactor supports the natural process of cells trying to maintain their environment to

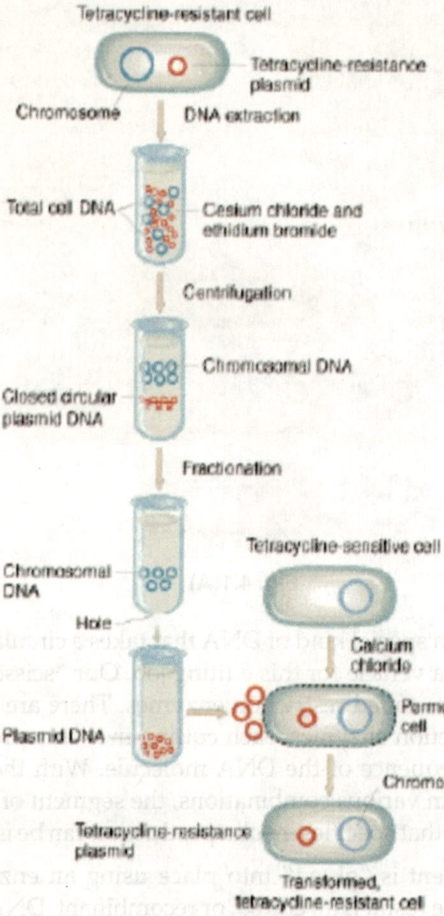

Fig. 4.1(B)

provide optimum growth conditions–by providing suitable conditions–temperature, pH, substrate, salts, vitamins, O2.

A primary goal of fermentation is the cost-effective production of desired products using high productivity techniques. Because most proteins are intracellularly accumulated. In recombinant *E. coli* and yeast productivity is proportional to the final cell-density and the specific productivity. Techniques for culturing *E. coli* or yeast have been developed to improve productivity and also to provide

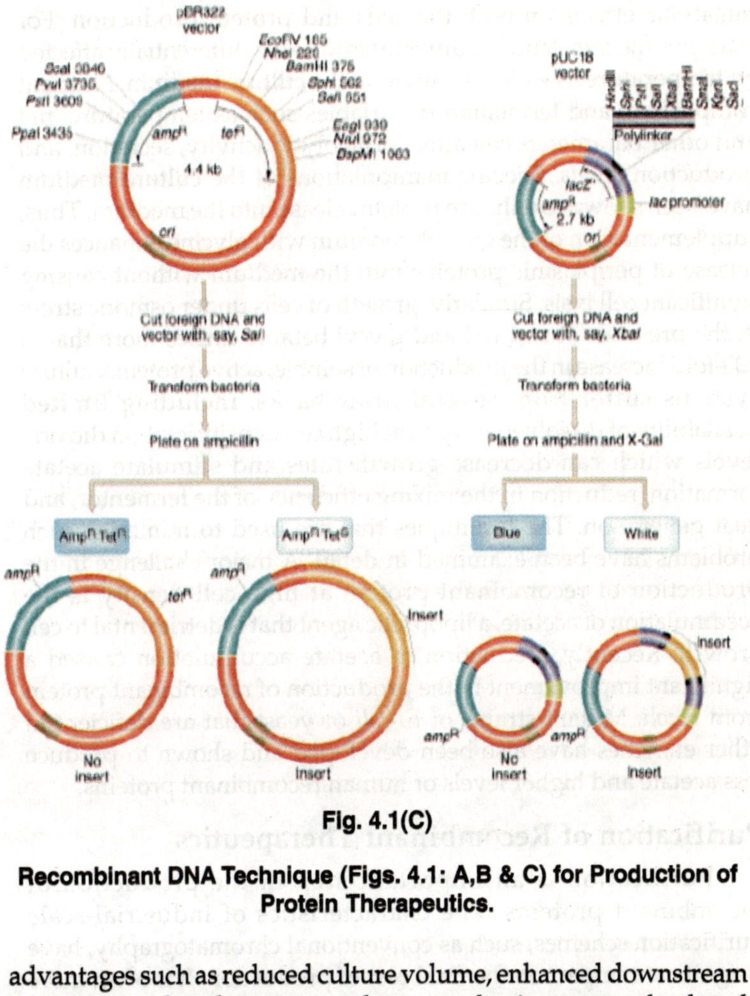

Fig. 4.1(C)

Recombinant DNA Technique (Figs. 4.1: A,B & C) for Production of Protein Therapeutics.

advantages such as reduced culture volume, enhanced downstream processing, reduced wastewater, lower production costs and reduced investment of equipment.

Protein production in *E. coli or yeast* can be increased significantly through the use of culture systems. These methods can achieve cell concentrations in excess of 100 g (dry cell weight)/liter and can provide cost-effective production of recombinant proteins. Detailed reviews of large-scale fermentation systems have been published. The composition of the cell growth medium must be carefully formulated and monitored, because it may have significant metabolic effects on both the cells and protein production. For example, the translation of different mRNAs is differentially affected by temperature as well as changes in the culture medium. Nutrient composition and fermentation variables such as temperature, pH and other parameters can affect proteolytic activity, secretion, and production levels. Specific manipulations of the culture medium have been shown to enhance protein release into the medium. Thus, supplementation of the growth medium with glycine enhances the release of periplasmic proteins into the medium without causing significant cell lysis. Similarly, growth of cells under osmotic stress in the presence of sorbitol and glycyl betaine causes more than a 400-fold increase in the production of soluble, active protein. Culture systems suffer from several draw-backs, including limited availability of dissolved oxygen at high cell density, carbon dioxide levels which can decrease growth rates and stimulate acetate formation, reduction in the mixing efficiency of the fermentor, and heat generation. The techniques that are used to minimize such problems have been examined in detail. A major challenge in the production of recombinant protein at high cell density is the accumulation of acetate, a lipophilic agent that is detrimental to cell growth. Recently, reduction in acetate accumulation caused a significant improvement in the production of recombinant protein from *E.coli*. Mutant strains of *E. coli* or yeast that are deficient in other enzymes have also been developed and shown to produce less acetate and higher levels of human recombinant proteins.

Purification of Recombinant Therapeutics

Purification is an important step in the production of recombinant proteins. The characteristics of industrial-scale purification schemes, such as conventional chromatography, have a significant impact on the final cost of production. It is often more efficient to use one of the available tags to 'fish out'the target protein. The purpose for which the protein will be used determines required degree for its purity and authenticity. To purify intracellularly produced proteins the cells are harvested and lysed, which naturally contributes to the complexity of the protein mixture. The advantage of intracellular versus secreted protein is the volume to be handled, *i.e.*, the secreted proteins usually exist diluted in the culture medium. Isolation of a desired protein from the medium follows the general scheme: (1) concentration by precipitation, ultrafiltration, batch adsorption or partition in an aqueous phase system (2) enrichment by chromatography or partition (3) high resolution purification: by chromatography and/or immuno adsorption (4)-final concentration. There are a variety of different methods which can be used to purify proteins, but only hromatographic purification methods such as affinity, ion exchange, reversed phase and gel filtration chromatography will be briefly describe here. Purification of a protein depends on this unique shape, which determines both its Biological Function and properties in solution.

Conventional Chromatography

Chromatographic methods (size exclusion, ion exchange, reversed phase, hydrophobic interaction and affinity based) can be utilized either in traditional, low pressure or highperformance liquid chromatography instrumentation. In addition to liquid-solid chromatography there is liquid-liquid chromatography which is analogous to gas-liquid chromatography. There are also many other types of chromatography methods *e.g.*, liquid adsorption chromatography, frontal chromatography, displacement chromatography covalent chromatography and membrane chromatography.

Ion Exchange Chromatography

Ion exchange chromatography (IEC) has been the most widely used technique for the isolation and purification of biological macromolecules since the 1950s. IEC is able to separate almost any type of charged molecules, from large proteins to small nucleotides and amino acids. The ion exchanger are insoluble solid matrices containing fixed ionogenic groups which bind reversibly to sample molecules (proteins, etc.). Desorption is then brought about by increasing the salt concentration or by altering the pH of the mobile phase. The two major classes of ion exhangers are cation exchangers and anion exchangers, having negatively and positively charged functional groups, respectively. Ion exchange containing diethyl aminoethyl (DEAE) or carboxymethyl (CM) groups are most frequently used.Since the protein is covered by a hydrophilic layer, electrostatic interactions have a major role in the retention of proteins. In addition to size, geometric form as well as hydrophopic and van der Walls interactions affect the separation. Nevertheless, the major property which govern the adsorption to an ion exchanger is the net surface charge of the protein. Since surface charge is the result of weak acidic and basic groups on proteins, separation is highly pH-dependent. The optimum pH range for IEC for many proteins is within 1 pH units of the isoelectric point. Many retention models have been examined but the complexity of the adsorption process for a protein to solid surfaces makes it difficult to construct physical models for the interactions. Gradient elution with increasing salt concentration is most commonly used in the IEC. The higher the net charge of the protein, the higher the ionic strength needed to bring about desorption. Thus, to optimize selectivity in ion exchange chromatography, the pH of the running buffer is chosen so that sufficiently large net charge differences among the sample components are created.

By summing the surface charges the net charge of the protein at a set pH, the protein will have negative, neutral, or positive charge. This is related to the pI of the protein. The method of ion exchange chromatography can be used to separate proteins with differing charges. Usually, the fixed charge groups are attached to cellulose fibers or beads.

Reversed Phase Chromatography

Reversed phase chromatography (RPC) can be utilized to separate compounds according to their hydrophobicity. Unlike many other methods RPC is able to separate closely related and structurally disparate substances, even at picomolar levels. In RPC, silica particles covered with chemically bonded hydrocarbon chains represent the lipophilic phase (C_2 to C_{18}), while an aqueous mixture of an organic solvent surrounding the particle represents the hydrophilic phase. Depending on the extractive power of the eluent, a greater or lesser part of the sample component will be retained reversibly by the lipid layer of the particles. The partitioning of the sample components between the two phases will depend on their respective solubility characteristics. Less hydrophobic components will end up primarily in the hydrophilic phase while more hydrophobic ones will be found in the lipophilic phase. This can be affected by the addition of an organic solvent which is soluble in the hydrophilic phase. Some commonly used organic solvents, in order of increasing hydrophobicity are methanol, propanol, acetonitrile, and etrahydrofuran. Separated components can be directly subjected to further analysis such as Edman sequencing or electrospray mass spectrometry. The ability of a stationary phase (lipophilic phase) to discriminate between two components is reflected by the volume between the peak maxima of the corresponding zones after passing through the column. Along with partitioning, mechanism adsorption operates at the interface between the mobile and the stationary phases. Thus, the retention of hydrophobic components will be greatly influenced by the thickness of the lipid layer. AC_{18} layer is able to accommodate more hydrophobic material than C_8 or C_2 ones. For hydrophilic components, changing from a C_{18} to a C_2 layer influences the separation very little since only the surface area of the lipid layer is active. The mobile phase can be considered as an aqueous solution of an organic solvent, the type and concentration of which determines the extractive power. Moreover,according to experimental data, components interact with the chromatographic surface in an orientation-specific manner. RPC has been utilized for purification of a variety of proteins and peptides *e.g.*, aprotinin, cytochrome C, bovine serum albumin, fibrinogen, insulin and lysosyme. Even though some proteins have been reported to maintain their native structure during RPC (*e.g.*, insulin, thyroid-stimulating hormone, growth hormone), in most cases denaturing conditions are required which might limit the use of RPC.

Gel Permeation Chromatography

The principle of gel permeation chromatography (GPC; size exclusion or gel filtration chromatography) is based on molecular volumes. Large molecules are excluded from the matrix, whereas intermediate size molecule can partly enter and only small molecules can freely enter the matrix. The porous three dimensional matrix acts as a steric barrier to solute molecules as they attempt to equilibrate with liquid inside and outside the bead. While purifying the protein GPC can also be used to estimate approximate molecular weights. Furthermore, gel filtration can be used for desalting or buffer changing when the fractionated size of the gel is small (*e.g.*, Bio-Gel 6, Sephadex G-25) allowing the protein to elute in the void volume. The choice of the appropriate column type depends on the molecular size and physical properties of the proteins to be separated. A fraction of the internal volume which is accessible to a solute molecule can be described by a constant Kd, which can be calculated with experimentally determined elution volumes. A column should be chosen so that separations occur in the linear part of the Kd vs. the molecular weight plot. However, it is practically impossible to adjust the pH and ionic strength so that the proteins are in an equal state, since at the isoelectric point the shape of globular and polymer coil proteins relieve compact and soft sphere, respectively. Furthermore, the ionic strength of the buffer used may affect the size of the proteins. Experiments with neutral dextrans and charged proteins showed that the effective protein size increases with decreasing ionic strength due to the reduction in electrostatic shielding. Thus, although GPC is viewed as size-based separation process, there is considerable evidence for the importance of electrostatic interactions as well. GPC has been used in the renaturation procedure. For example heterodimeric platelet-derived growth factor was purified from inclusion bodies after denaturation with Gdn-HCl. Renaturation of this growth factor involved folding into an active heterodimeric form during GPC while circumventing aggregation observed when refolding was carried out by dilution.

Affinity Chromatography

Affinity chromatography together with recombinant DNA-technology offers a simple and fast technique to purify proteins to high purity with a single purification step. Fusion can be made on either side or both sides of the target gene depending on specific application, but the majority of fusion proteins place the tag at the N-terminus of the protein. Genetic manipulation of the protein can be used to form a cleavage site, which helps to remove the affinity tag after purification thereby resulting in an intact protein. Although affinity chromatography can be used for laboratory-scale purification, its utilization on a preparative scale can represent a major cost for the final protein product. Successful separation by affinity chromatography requires that a biospecific ligand is available, and that it is covalently attached to a chromatographic bed material. It is important that the biospecific ligand (antibody, enzyme, or receptor protein) retains its specific binding affinity for the substance of interest (antigen, substrate, or hormone). These interactions typically have high affinities (Kd < 10-6 M), yet are reversible when conditions are changed. Due to the specificity of this recognition, it is often possible to obtain 100-, 1,000- or even 100,000-fold increases in purity of a protein sample. The packing material used, called the affinity matrix, must be inert and easily modified. Agarose is the most common substance used as a matrix, in spite of its relative high costs. The ligands, or "affinity tails", that are inserted into the matrix can be genetically engineered to possess a specific affinity. In a process similar to ion exchange chromatography, the desired molecules adsorb to the ligands on the matrix until esorption is carried out *e.g.*, with a high salt concentration, a competition reaction (*e.g.*, imidazole), strong chelating agents and/or low pH. Fouling of the matrix can occur when a large number of impurities are present, therefore, this type of chromatography is usually implemented late in the process. In addition to most common affinity chromatography utilizing HPLC, there are also other techniques which involve affinity, such as affinity precipitation, affinity partitioning of proteins using aqueous two-phase system, foam fractionation and dye ligand chromatography.

Affinity Tags

To date, a large number of different fusion partners that range in size from one amino acid to whole proteins capable of selective interaction with ligand immobilized onto a chromatography matrix, have been described. Although a multitude of systems have been introduced, no single affinity fusion partner is ideal for all expression or purification systems. Some of the most commonly used tags are reviewed below and listed in Table 1.

In 1975 Porath and co-workers introduced a method based on the interaction between the side chains of certain amino acids, especially histidines, on a protein surface and immobilized transition metal ions. Immobilized metal affinity chromatography (IMAC) systems have three basic components: an electron donor group, a solid support and a metal ion. The metal ion (usually Ni2+, Co2+, Cu2+ or Zn2+) is restrained in a coordination complex where it still retains significant affinity towards macromolecules. The use of polyhistidine tags has been demonstrated in a wide range of host cells including *E. coli, P.pastoris,* insect cells as well as in mammalian cells. IMAC is usually performed under nondenaturing conditions, but it is also compatible with non-ionic detergents allowing highly denaturing conditions with urea and guanidium-HCl. Also an organic solvent (isopropanol) can be used to increase the purification efficiency. The elution is usually performed by competition with imidazole, lowering pH, or by adding strong chelating agents. IMAC is particularly suitable for preparative group fractionation of complex extracts and biofluids, but can also be used in the high-performance mode. Regardless of the relatively small size of the his-tag, is has been reported recombinant proteins. Maltose binding protein (MBP) from *E.coli* is frequently used as a fusion partner for proteins. MBP (40 kDa) is a periplasmic protein and thereby can be employed to induce the secretion into the periplasm. A mixture of cellulose and starch can be utilized as a ligand and elution can be achieved in the presence of maltose. MBP has reported to increase the solubility of the fusion protein and it has been successfully used as a C-terminal fusion partner.Glutathione S-Transferase (GST) -fusion vectors were first reported. GSTs are a family of enzymes that can transfer sulfur from glutathione to substances such as nitro and halogenated compounds, leading to their detoxication. GST fusion proteins are bound to immobilized glutathione reduced glutathione. Since GST is a relatively large tag (26 kDa), in many cases it is preferable to remove it by engineering a specific cleavage site. GST can also be utilized under denaturing conditions. However, a possible complication associated with this system is the use of reduced glutathione for elution, since it can affect target proteins containing disulfides. Staphylococcal protein A is a immunoglobulin-binding receptor on the surface of the gram-positive bacterium *Staphylococcus aureus*. Protein A (30 kDa) and its derivative Z shows a specific affinity for the Fc-region of immunoglobulin G. Protein A consists of five repetitive homologous domains (A-E), and each of these domains alone is capable of binding to IgG. The structure of the B domain (from which Z has been derived) has been determined, revealing that the N- and C-termini of the three-helix bundle structure are solvent exposed, which is supposed to favor an independent folding of the target protein. Analysis of different repeats of Z showed that there is no advantage in using more than two domains. Protein A is secretion competent and fusion proteins can be secreted to the *E. coli* periplasm and in some cases also to the culture medium. Protein A has been reported to be highly soluble and capable of renaturation after being subjected to denaturants such as urea and guanidium HCl. The need for low pH for elution can be circumvented by the use of competitive elution strategies based on engineered competitor proteins. Like protein A, Staphylococcal protein G, is a receptor present on the surface of certain strains of *Streptococci*. Protein G is a bifunctional protein having structurally separate regions for affinity to serum albumin and IgG. The serum albumin binding region has three helix-bundle domains, very similar to that of protein A. Elution

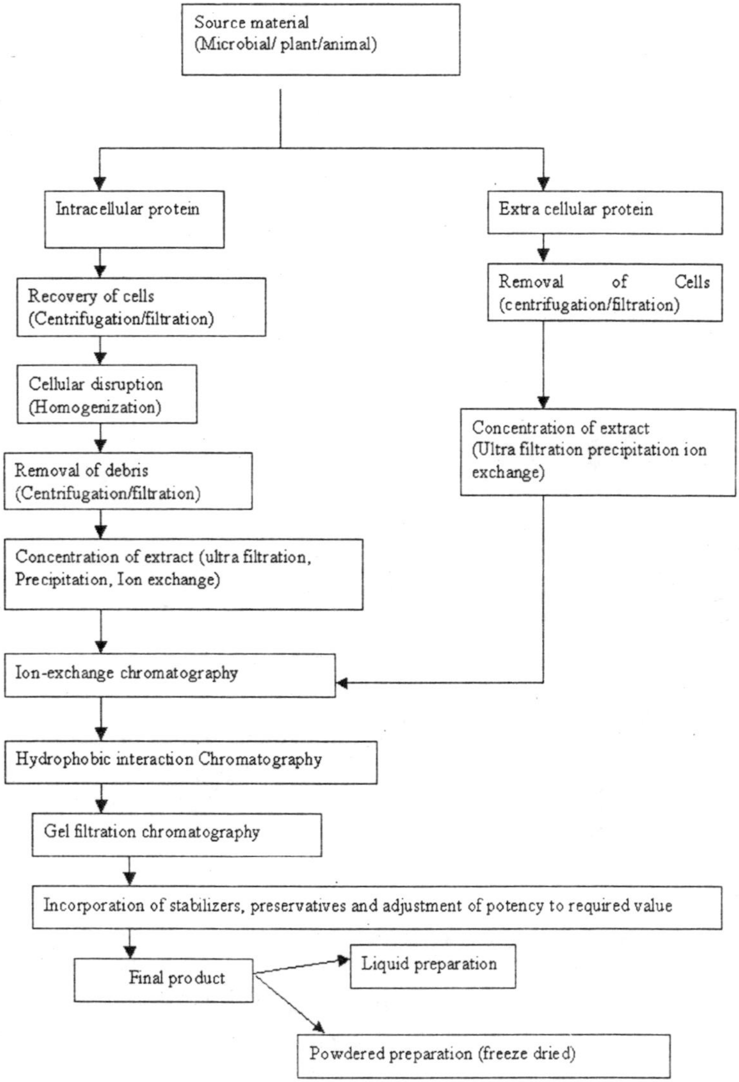

Fig. 4.2: Purification Strategies for Protein Based Drugs.

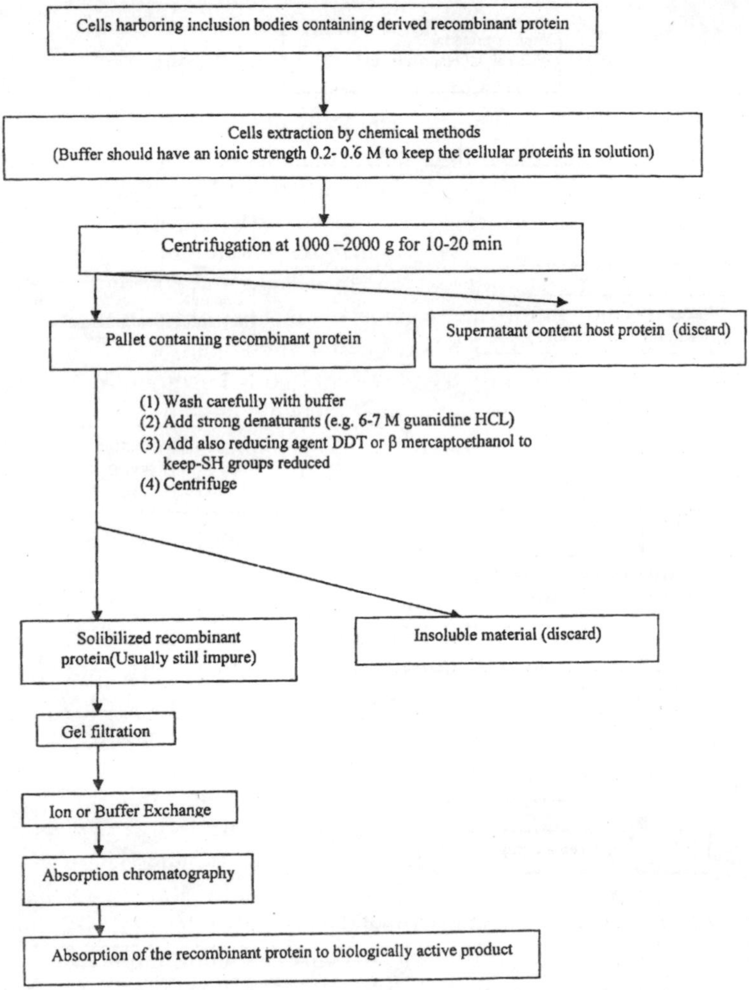

Fig. 4.3: A Schematic Procedure to Purify Recombinant Proteins in *E.coli* as Inclusion Bodies.

from a column is usually achieved with low pH or by alternative methods such as high pH, lithium diiodosalisylate and heat. Protein G or different parts of the albumin binding domain have been used as affinity tags in protein expressed either intracellularly or as secreted proteins.

E. coil pest containing precursors

↓ At the extant 25% of total cellular protein

→ **Supernatant (Discard)**

↓ Homogenized in aquas buffer at pH 8.0 and centrifuged

Pellet

↓ Washed in 3M GuHCL

Pellet containing insoluble precursors (=75% of total proteins)

↓ Added 75% HCOOH and treated with CNBr

Almost quantities yield of pro-insulin monomers (30-40 mg /g dry cell mass)

↓ Sulfotolysis with sodium sulfate and sodium tetrathionate in 6 M GuHCL

Pro-insulin analog (PIA) S-sulfonate

↓ Purification by anion exchange chromatography with 25% formaldehyde pH 8.5 and eluted with Nacl gradient (2 g PIA was proceed in a 5 X15 cm column)

Pure pro-insulin analog s-sulfonate

↓ Dilution of S-sulphonate to ,5.0 mg/ml and incubation at pH 9.3 3X molar excess glutathione over [-SO_3] for 24 hr at 4^0C

Refolded pro-insulin analog s-sulfonate

↓ Liberated from contaminants by hydrophobic interaction chromatography on octyl-Sepharose equilibrated with 0.4 M CH_3COOK at pH 7.3 and eluted with isopropanol (linear gradient 0-20%, V/V); A 5 X 15 cm column proceed ~ 1 g protein

Nearly homologous folded PIA with corrected disulfide bonds

↓ Brief exposure to trypsin and carboxypeptidase B at pH 7.3 and 25^0C

Insulin (60-65% of starting PIA) + contaminants

↓ Preparative RP-HPLC

Pure, biologically active Insulin

Fig. 4.4: Purification of Insulin Expressed by a Poly Pro-insulin Construct

(Ref. R Seetharam and SK Sharma (ed): Purification and analysis of recombinant protein (2000) Marcel Deker Inc. New York.3-28 pp)

Culture supernatant containing Protein (40C)

↓

Affinity chromatography column (5 X 10 cm) on Zn + chelating agarose equilibrated with 20 mM Tris-HCL pH 7.5, 1M Nacl, 0.01 % Tween 80, Elution with 0-50 mM imidazole gradient in the above Buffer

↓

Affinity chromatography column (0.9 X 25 cm) on concanavalin A-garose equilibrated with 10 mM Tris-HCL pH 7.5, 1M Nacl, 0.01 % Tween-80, Elution with 0-0.2 M a-d-methylmanoside and 0-1 M KSCN

↓

Gel filtration on sephadex G-150 column (2.5 X 90 cm) equilibrated with 10 mM sodium phosphate buffer, pH 7.5, 1.6 M KSCN, 0.01% Tween 80

↓

Dialysis against 0.15 M Nacl + 0.01 % Tween 80 (V/V) t PA Yield (near about 50%) and spesific activity 90,000IV/mg

Fig. 4.5: Purification of Tissue Plasminogen Activator (tPA) from Human Melanoma Cells.

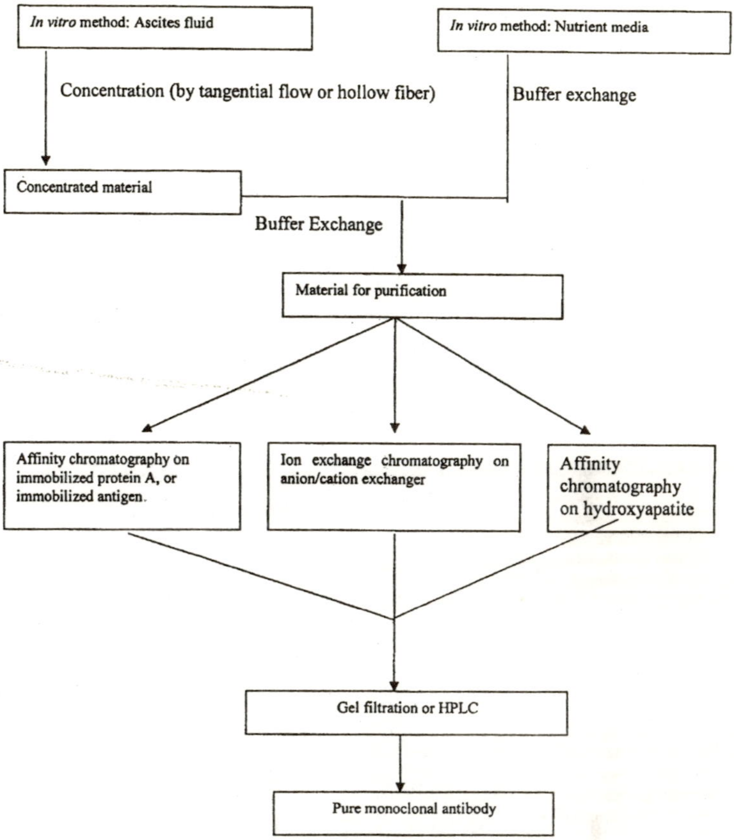

Fig. 4.6: A Scheme for Monoclonal Antibody Purification.

The eventual objective of producing a desired prote through an economical purification is influenced by a variety of factors. However, maximizing production heterologous proteins for commercial application is still an art. To perform this, chose of proper chromatography techniques is necessary. So, chromatography have a significant importance to get maximum label of purification and to make cheaper cost of production.

Chapter 5

Quality Control and Characterization

After the production, you need to characterize your protein. There are some methods for characterization. The methods are as follows:

1. Sodium Dodecyl Sulfate–Poly Acrylamide Gel Electrophoresis
2. Bradford/Lowry Assays (Concentration)
3. UV Light Spectroscopy (Concentration)
4. Amino Acid Analysis (Composition)
5. Amino Acid Sequencing (Primary Structure)
6. Optical Rotary Dispersion (2 D Structure)
7. Circular Dichroism (2 D Structure)
8. FTIR (2 D Structure)
9. Atomic Force Microscopy (Tertiary (3D) and Quaternary (4D) Structure Characterization)
10. Biological activity determination or Bio assay

The highlight of all above methods are following:

Sodium Dodecyl Sulfate–Poly Acrylamide Gel Electrophoresis

SDS-PAGE (denaturing-PAGE)

Separate proteins according to their size.

SDS is a detergent. Detergents have affinities for hydrophobic regions of proteins.

SDS is a negatively charged detergent.

Mixing detergent with a soluble protein will lead to denaturation of the protein as the hydrophobic buried regions of the protein are solubilized (dissolved).

In the case of SDS you end up with a linearized (denatured) polypeptide chain, coated with negative charges in such a way that the magnitude of the charge is proportional to the size of the protein. All proteins coated with SDS will have the same structure and the same charge density and differ only in their overall length (size).

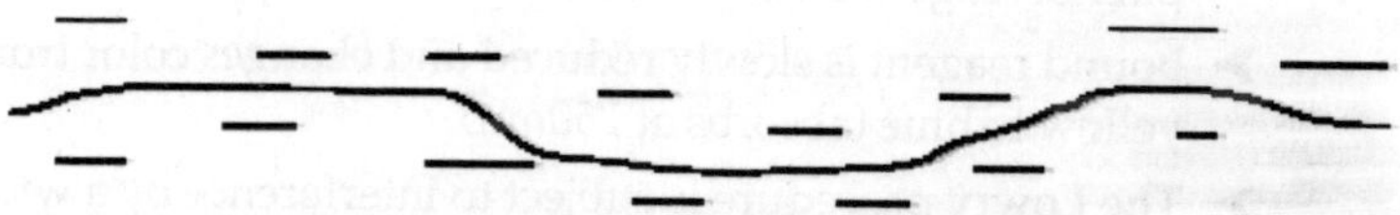

Fig. 5.1: Chare density of SDS

You might want to add a reducing agent (dithiothreitol or 2-mercatoethanol) to break disufide bridges that otherwise prevent the linearization of the polypeptide backbone.

If you put these denatured/reduced proteins, that all maintain identical negative charge:mass ratios, into an electric field they will all move toward the positive pole at the same rate.

If you put a porous gel system (sieve) between the protein and the positive pole, smaller protein will be able to move through the pores faster than the big proteins, so you will get separation of your proteins based on size.

Proteins in the gels are stained with Coomassie Blue for visualization.

Non-denaturing and/or non-reducing gels can be run as well.

Quantitation of Total Protein in a Given Sample

Lowry Method (**Lowry** ***et al., J. Biol. Chem.*** **193: 265-275 (1951)**)

➤ Under alkaline conditions, copper complexes with protein.

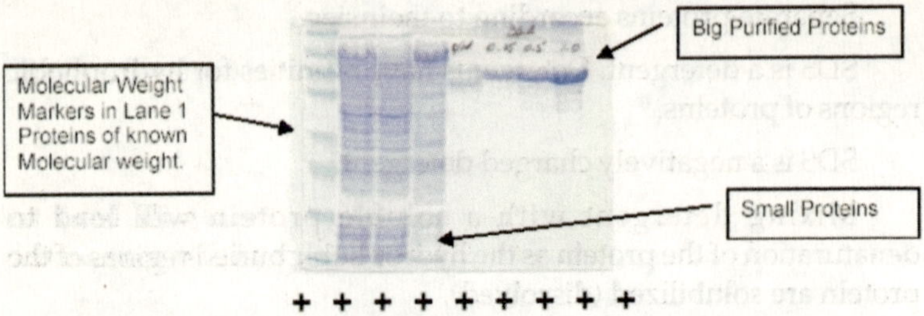

Fig. 5.2: Sodium Dodecyl Sulfate – Poly Acrylamide Gel Electrophoresis

- When folin phenol reagent (phospho-molybdic-phosphotungstic mixed acid reagent) is added, the Folin-phenol reagent binds to the copper bound protein.
- bound reagent is slowly reduced and changes color from yellow to blue (absorbs at 750nm).
- The Lowry procedure is subject to interference by a wide variety of chemicals.

***Bradford Method* (Bradford, *Anal. Biochem.* 72: 248, (1976)**

- The Bradford protein assay depends upon the change in absorbance in Coomassie Blue G-250 upon binding of protein (changed compound absorbs at 595nm).
- Unlike the Lowry procedure, the Bradford assay is not susceptible to interference by a wide variety of chemicals present in samples.

How to Determine Protein Concentration by Lowry or Bradford Methods

1. Using a standard protein such as Bovine Serum Albumin (BSA), make up 5 samples over a range of known concentrations: eg) 0.1mg/ml, 0.2mg/ml, 0.5 mg/ml, 1.0mg/ml, 2.0mg/ml.
2. Carry out the Lowry or Bradford assay as described above.
3. Measure absorbance readings (A750 or A595 depending on the method) for the known BSA concentration samples. Make a plot of Absorbance versus Concentration.
4. Perform assay on unknown sample and use standard plot to determine protein concentration.

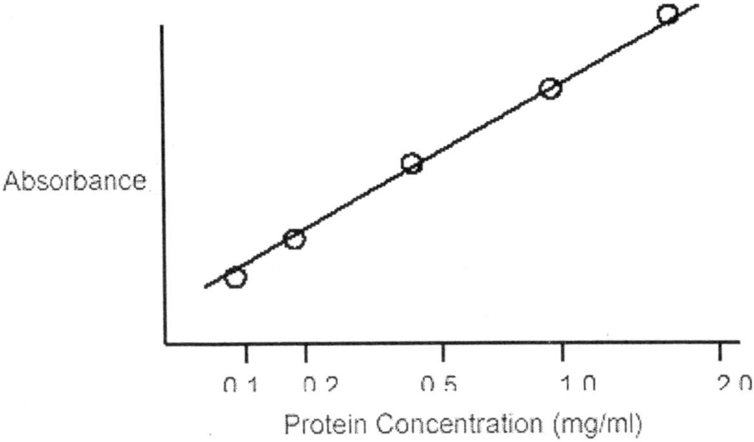

Fig. 5.3: Plot for determine the protein concentration

Quantitation by UV Light Spectroscopy

The aromatic ring structures of tryptophan and tyrosine show significant absorption of light at 280nm wavelength. Proteins that contain these amino acids can be quantitated by UV Spectroscopy. Although the protein must be pure.

According to the formula:

$$A = \varepsilon CL$$

A is the absorbance at 280nm.

C is the concentration of the protein (M)

L is the pathlength (cm)

ε is the 'extinction coefficient' or molar absorption coefficient ($M^{-1} cm^{-1}$)

ε can be calculated from the sequence (using computer programs) or from experimental determination

The Y-axis on any elution profile would have been an A280 value.

Sample Problem

If you measure an A280 value of 0.5 for a purified protein of known extinction coefficient (42,000 M-1 cm-1) using a cuvette with a 1cm pathlength, what is you concentration?

$$A = \varepsilon CL$$

$$C = A/\varepsilon L$$

$$C = 0.5/(42{,}000)$$

$$C = 1.2x10\text{-}5\ M$$

Peptide Bonds Absorb light at 210nm.

The Peptide bond is the covalent bond that exists between the C-terminus of one amino acid and the N-terminus of the next one in a chain of amino acids.

If your protein lacks aromatic side chains A210 readings can be made instead.

Amino Acid Analysis (Composition)

Refers to the determination of the relative amounts of each of the 20 different amino acids in a given protein.

Step1: Hydrolysis

The polypeptide chain is hydrolyzed into individual amino acids by exposure to 6M HCl at 110°C for 24-72 hours.

Step 2: Separation

Ion exchange Chromatography is used to separate the amino acid mixture. At pH 2.0, all amino acids bind to sulfonated polystyrene resin. Amino acids are eluted with high pH and high ionic strength.

Step 3: Quantitation

The purified amino acid fractions are mixed with ninhydrin, which reacts with the amino acids and produces a blue purple color that absorbs at 570nm, and allows quantitation by $A=\varepsilon CL$.

Alternative Method

After Step1, the amino acids are derivatized by reaction with phthaldehyde + 2-mercaptoethanol to make fluorescent compounds which can be separated by HPLC.

AAA Issues

Tryptophan is destroyed under these conditions. Tryptophan content is determined separately by alkaline or enzymatic hydrolysis or determined by spectral methods.

Serine and Threonine are slowly destroyed with half lives of 50-100 hours. Accurate quantitation requires detection over time (24, 48 and 72 hours) and extrapolation to time 0.

Cyteine, 20% of cysteine are destroyed after 24hours. Cysteine can be converted to Cysteic Acid before hydrolysis and then they are stable.

Protein-SH + H-C-COOH Protein-SO3⁻

Valine and Isoleucine are beta carbon branched amino acids and their side chains sterically shield the acid attack on the peptide linkage. Need longer time 48-72 hours.

Asparigine, Aspartate, Glutamine and Glutamate, Upon acid hydrolysis Asparagine and Glutamine are converted to Aspartate and Glutamate and they are quantitated as ASX (total ASP and ASN) and GLX (total GLU and GLN).

The total amount of ASN and GLN may be determined by quantitation of released ammonia. Alternatively enzymatic hydrolysis may be used.

Overall you get the relative ratios of the amino acids present in a given proteins.

To quantitate the precise numbers you must know the molecular weight of the protein as well as the amount of protein total that was hydrolyzed.

Generally with the intrinsic errors in the protocol the calculated molar ratios are rarely close to actual values.

Amino-Acid Sequencing

Refers to determination of the sequence or order of amino acids in a peptide or protein.

The amino acid sequence is also referred to as the Primary Structure of a protein.

Amino Terminal Residue

Generally all methods involve chemical labeling of the amino-terminus, hydrolyzing the protein into constituent amino acids and then determination of which amino acid type is labeled.

Two Common Methods

Following acid hydrolysis the labeled amino acids are identified by their yellow color in the fluoro-2,4-dinitrobenzene procedure and by fluresence when the dansyl chloride is used.

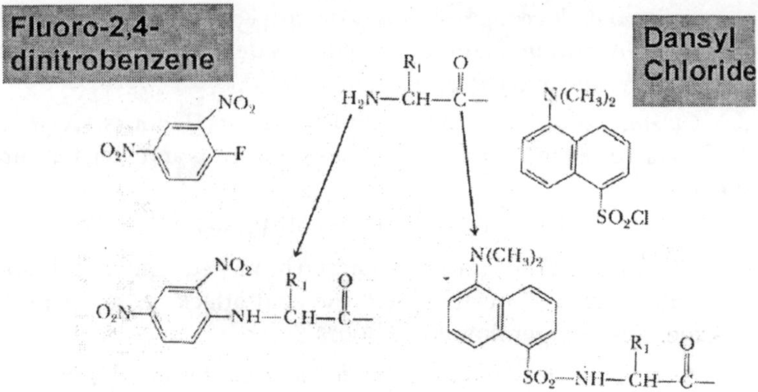

Fig. 5.4: Amino Terminal Residue

A Related Procedure

Reaction with Cyanate

This Cyanate reaction forms the Basis of the Edman Degredation used in automated protein sequencing instruments.

Edman Degredation

In the Edman degredation only the amino-terminal derivatized amino acid is removed from the polypeptide chain, allowing for continuous cycling of the reaction to identify sequential amino acids, rather than just the amino terminal residue.

The sequence of up to 60 Amino Acids can be determined by the Edman Degradation under favorable conditions.

Errors are cumulative.

Any unreacted amino acid will not be removed by hydrolysis and will contribute additional background to subsequent cycles.

Total Protein Sequencing

Most proteins are longer than 60 amino acids. In order to obtain the complete sequence of a protein the following steps are required.

1. Fragmentation of the polypeptide chain into smaller peptides (20-30 amino acids).

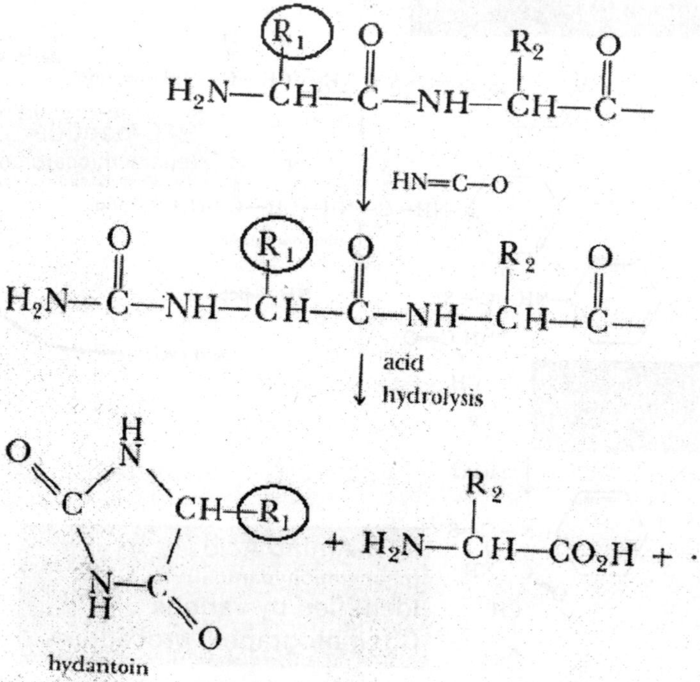

Fig. 5.5: Reaction with Cyanate

2. Isolation and purification of these smaller peptides
3. Determination of the amino acid sequence by Edman Degradation

   This will get you the complete sequence of each peptide, but you have to determine the overall order of the peptides that make up the protein.
4. Repeat Steps 1-3, using an alternative fragmentation method that will yield a second set of peptides that will over lap with the first set to determine the order of the peptides.

Methods of Fragmentation include

CNBr–Cyanogen Bromide Cleavage–cleaves the chain on the carbonyl side of Methionine Rsidues.

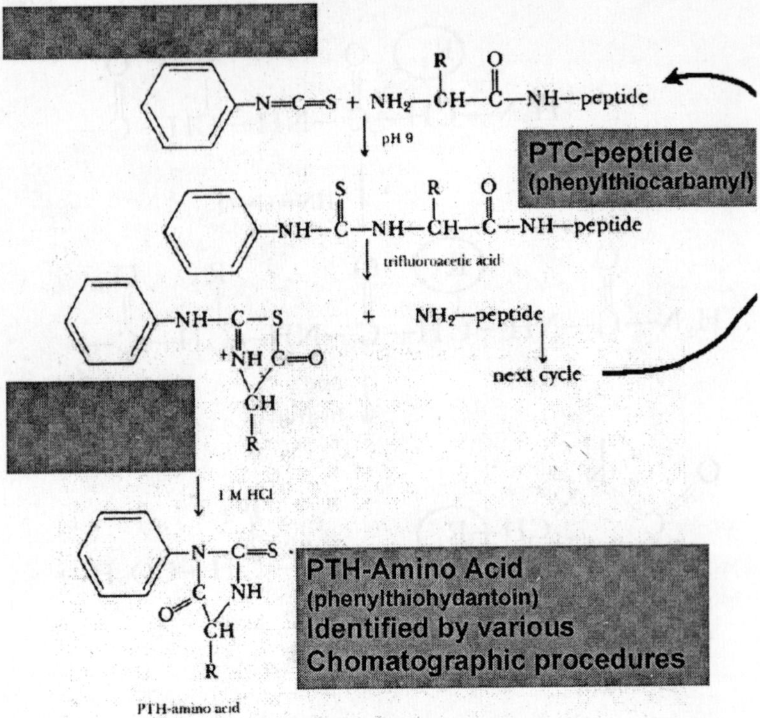

Fig. 5.6: Edman Degredation

Enzymatic Cleavage–

Eg: Trypsin–cleaves peptide bonds on the carbonyl side of Arg and Lys residues.

Eg: Chymotrypsin–cleaves peptide bonds on the carbonyl side of Phe, Tyr and Trp

Eg: Elastase–cleaves peptide bonds on the carbonyl side of Gly and Ala.

Carboxy-Terminal Identification:

Hydrazinolysis

Not good for sequential analysis. Only applicable to determintation of the absolute terminal carboxy-amino acid.

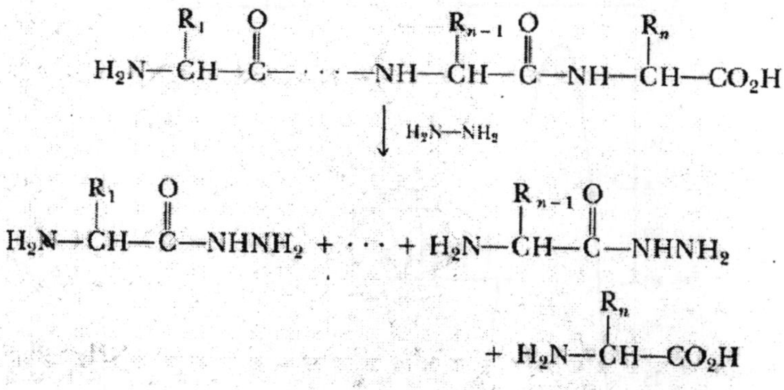

Fig. 5.7: Hydrazinolysis

Optical Rotary Dispersion (Characterization of Secondary (2D) Structure)

Helix, B-sheet and randomn coil content

Optical Rotary Dispersion (ORD)

Based on optical activity of polypeptides due to the asymmetric centers and conformations of L-amino acids.

1. The asymmetry causes them to interact differently right and left circularly polarized light.
2. If the two beams of light travel at different speed through the molecule the polarized light will be rotated.
3. ORD measures the dependence of this rotation on the wavelength of light.
4. The ORD pattern is dependent upon the Structure content of the polypeptide chain.

Poly-Lysine:

Low and Neutral pH = Randomn Coil

High pH= Helical,

High temperature = B-

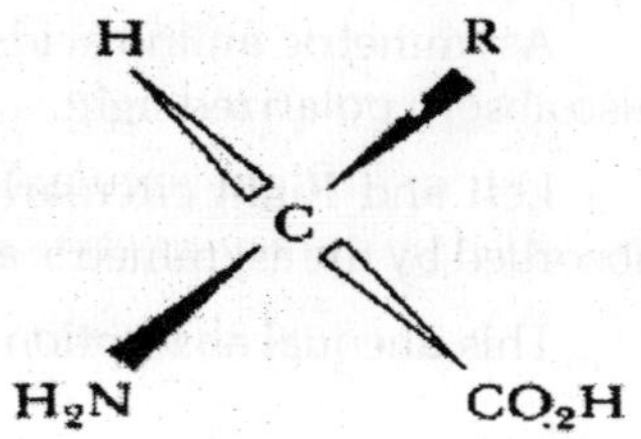

Fig. 5.8

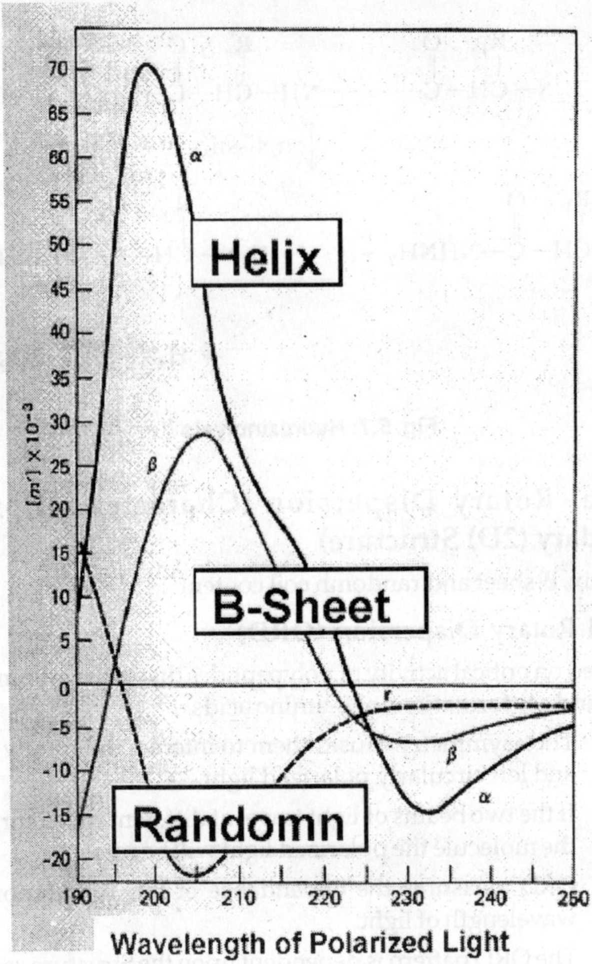

Fig. 5.9(a): Circular Dichroism

Circular Dichroism (CD)

Asymmetric amino acids not only rotate polarized light, but also absorb polarized light.

Left and Right circularly polarized light will be unequally absorbed by the asymmetric amino acids.

This unequal absorption is call circular dichroism.

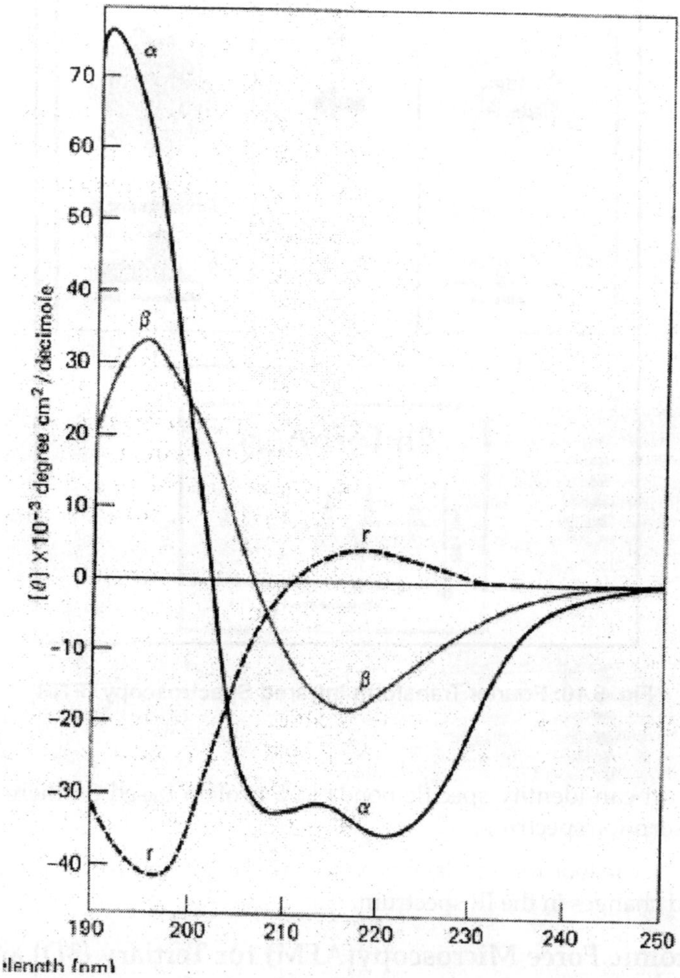

Fig. 5.9(b): Circular Dichroism

Fourier Transform Infrared Spectroscopy (FTIR)

FTIR is sensitive to bond vibrational frequencies. Bonds vibrating at certain frequencies will absorb energy in the infrared range.

The exact wavelength at which a bond will absorb depends on the exact frequency at which it is vibrating.

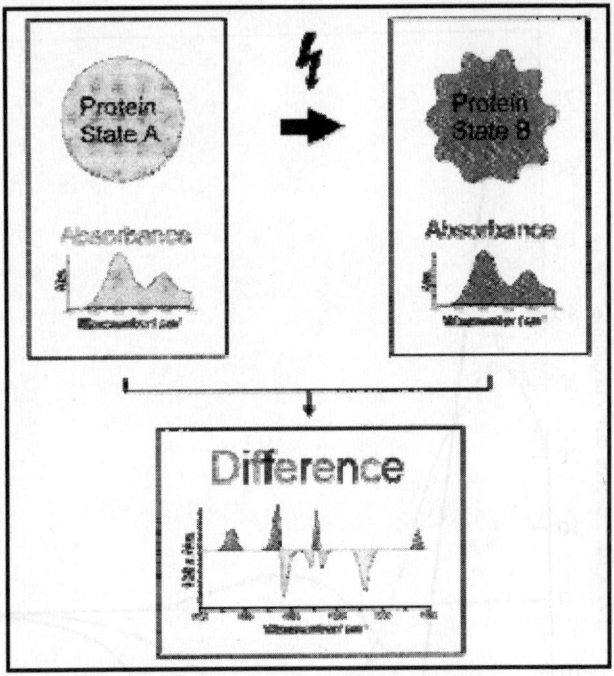

Fig. 5.10: Fourier Transform Infrared Spectroscopy (FTIR)

It can identify specific bonds in a protein based on there IR absorption spectrum.

It can look for correlations between different states of the protein and changes in the IR spectrum.

Atomic Force Microscopy(AFM) for Tertiary (3D) and Quarternary (4D) Structure Characterization

Basic Concept

A sharp probe is mounted at the end of a flexible cantilever, and then scans the topology (surface) of a layer. When the probe hits a 'hill' in the layer it is forced up and the flexible cantilever is flexed up. The up and down motion of the lever is monitored.

This system is sensitive to Angstrom resolution.

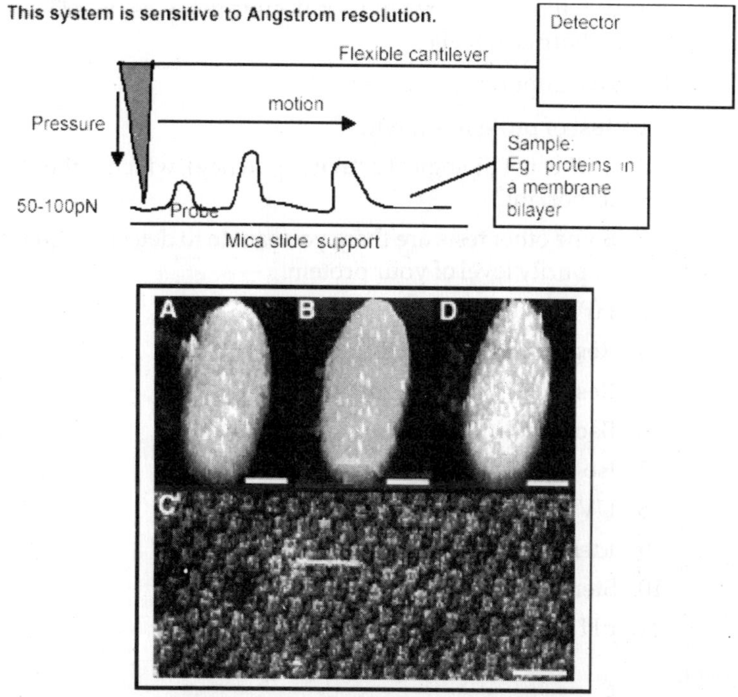

Fig. 5.11: Concept of Atomic Force Microscopy

Biological Activity Determination or Bio Assay

For therapeutics it is necessary to determine the biological activity. In case of new proteins you have to determine with a new method. We can give the following example-

The biological activity of recombinant GCSF demonstrated *in vivo* with rat. Neutropenia in normal mice was induced by a single combined intraperitoneal injection of 130 mg/kg of cyclophosphamide (CPA), 4.5 mg/kg of doxorubicin (DXR) and 1mg/kg of vincristine (VCR) into ICR mice on day 0. The purified G-CSF (100m/kg/day) will be subcutaneously administrated for 5 consecutive days starting 1 day after injection of anticancer agents. The change of neutrophils will be observed for two weeks.

The biological activity of recombinant salmon calcitonin (sCT) demonstrate *in vivo* with rat hypercalcemic assay as described in the British Pharmacopoeia

The most important tests are:

1. Test of protein contents
2. The test of biological activity (potency), which is the most important.

   Some other tests are there you can do to detect the quality or purity level of your protein:
3. HPLC purity
4. Residual bacterial DNA
5. Residual bacterial protein
6. Bacterial Endo toxin
7. Iso-electric point
8. UV spectrophotometer analysis
9. Identification test
10. Sterility test
11. pH Measurement

Chapter 6

Transgenic Technology: Another Methods of Production

Transgenic technology is a technique to introduce a foreign gene (a recombinant DNA) into the nucleus of an embryo by microinjection, creating a transgenic animal that secretes proteins (called transgenic proteins) in milk or blood. The transgenic proteins are purified, tested and become the therapeutic drugs. With this technology, many human proteins such as antibodies, enzymes, plasma proteins, fusion proteins are developed and producing; now many of them are in clinical trials and preclinical studies. These human protein may replace the bovine or porcine derived proteins because of the safety concerns about pathogens and allergic reactions. The advantages of using transgenic technology compared to mammalian cell culture technology are low-cost and ease of scale-up. Thus the transgenic animals are considered as a bioreactor for the production of biopharmaceutical products in the future. Here are the examples of transgenic proteins in clinical trials.

Human proteins for therapeutic use have been produced by extraction from tissues and plasma and by recombinant technology from mammalian and microbial cells that oftentimes sacrificed cost effectiveness for a large scale production of pure, native and stable proteins. As transgenic technology makes considerable progress, so called non-scientefically "animal factory" has drawn much attention for the production of native human proteins in a large and economically feasible scale. Success is now coming in.

Take antithrombin III for example. It was produced at 8-10 g/L in transgenic goat milk (Genzyme Transgenics) that was similar to that in transgenic mice for research purpose. Approximate productivity comparison with CHO (Chinese hamster ovary) cells is as follows for 10 kg of ATIII: goat milk 2100 liters (7 goats, lactation 150 days, 16 g/2 L/day, 60 % recovery); CHO cells 17000 liters (batch, 10-day cycle, 1 g/L, 60% recovery). Purification of the protein was much easier from goat milk with only a few steps than from cell culture. The production of similar level was also achieved for albumin and monoclonal antibodies. Economically feasible cost for human albumin production is ca $1/g so far by extraction from plasma and recombinant technology from yeast. This is now achievable by transgenic technology.

Most advanced in "animal factory" are Genzyme Transgenics (USA; goat and cow for ATIII, human serum albumin, tissue plasminogen activator, monoclonal antibodies), PPL Therapeutics (England; sheep and cow for alpha 1 protease inhibitor/cystic fibrosis, alpha-lactoalbunin, factor IX) and Pharming (Holland; cow and rabbit for alpha-glucosidase/glycogen storage disease, type II). Typically and Technically, a strong milk promoter (bovine alpha casein: 10 mg/ml, goat beta casein: 16 mg/ml, sheep lactoglobulin: 3 mg/ml) is selected for transgene expression and the expression vector is microinjected into fertilized eggs that are transferred into recipient female. Offsprings are tested for the transgene. Transgenic animals mate. Then milk transgenic female. In the farm for "animal factories", GAP (Good Agricultural Practice) is observed according to FDA's "Points to Consider in the Manufacture and Testing of Therapeutic Products for Human Use Derived from Transgenic Animals. Thus, for example, virus and scrapie validation is carried out for the transgenic products.

SMI (Sumitomo Metal Industries) Genzyme now plans to carry out a clinical trial in Japan of recombinant antithrombin III produced from goat milk as it demonstrated safety and efficacy of the treatment of 30 patient of artery bypass surgery in the USA. Plasma-derived ATIII (now $75 million in Japan per year for disseminated intravascular coagulation) may be replaced by transgenic counterpart if the trials are successful.

Similarly, transgenic monoclonal antibodies are quite promising as they may replace humanized mAbs for therapeutic use. The possibility of immune reaction to humanized antibodies depends on the extent of humanization and it has to wait till clinical trials of such mAbs to assess immunogenicity. Humanization, however, has made several mAbs real therapeutic possibilities for breast cancer (HER2/neu/c-erbB-2: Herceptin, Genentech), Crohn's disease (Avakine, Centocor), non-Hodgkins lymphoma (Rituxan, Genentech, approved 11/97), and several others for leukemia, head and neck cancer, heart disease, asthma and transplant rejection. So mAbs are coming back after a long spell of disappointment. It is now most likely that transgenic technology gradually replaces hybridization technique for mAb production. This is especially useful for the production of native human mABs with least immeunogenicity and better characteristics of stability and permeability

Table 6.1

Protein name	*Source*	*Application*	*Company*
Alpha-1-antitrypsin	Sheep	Cystic fibrosis, Emphysema	PPL Therapeutics
Antithrombin III (a plasma protein)	Goat	Antithrombin III deficiency	Genzyme Transgenics
Human alpha-glucosidase (an enzyme)	Rabbit	Pompe's disease	Pharming Group
Human collagen type II (a structural protein)	Chicken	Rheumatoid arthritis	Pharming Group
PRO 542 (a fusion protein)	Goat	HIV disease	Genzyme Transgenics
Remicade (a monolonal antibody)	Goat	Grohn's disease, Rheumatoid arthritis	Genzyme Transgenics

This procedure has now been successful in both pigs and cows. Among animals, the pig has a number of advantages. Its gestation period is only four months. At 12 months of age the pig is fertile and produces large litter sizes (usually 10 to 12 piglets). A lactating pig/cow produces 300 liters (about 315 quarts) of milk in a year. The procedure is carried out as follows:

1. The DNA fragment (gene) that codes for the needed human protein is isolated.

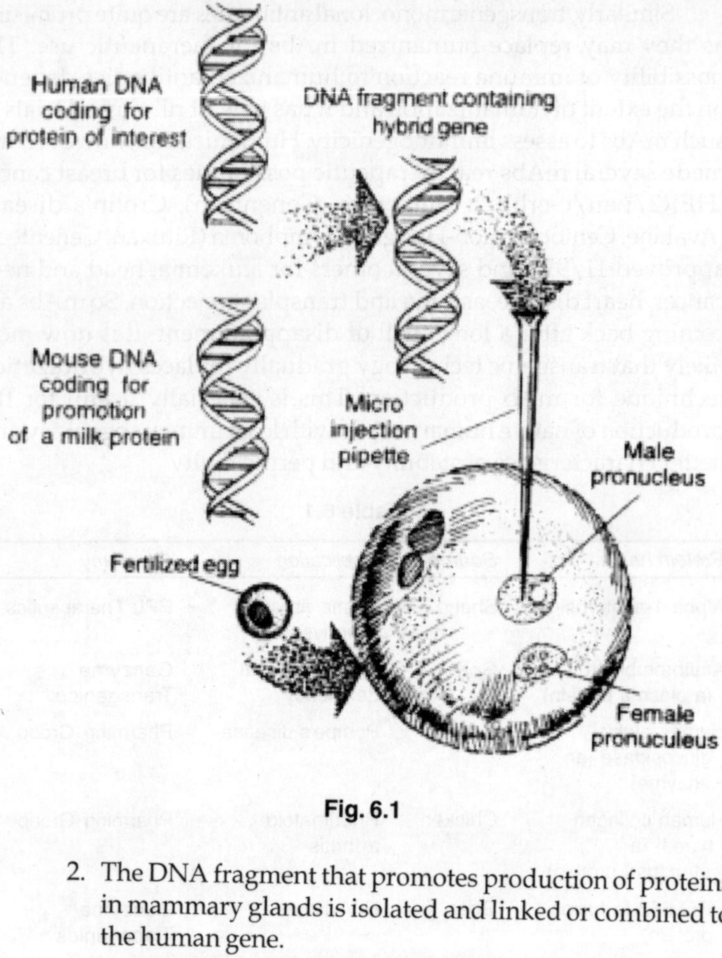

Fig. 6.1

2. The DNA fragment that promotes production of proteins in mammary glands is isolated and linked or combined to the human gene.
3. Fertilized eggs from a donor pig or cow are obtained.
4. The human DNA is injected into an egg in the region of the male pronucleus (DNA from the sperm before it unites with DNA of the egg) using a very slim micro pipette. The human DNA is thus incorporated into the pig or cow nuclear DNA.
5. The egg is implanted in the uterus of another pig or cow and develops into a newborn female pig or cow .
6. The desired protein is isolated from the milk of the female pig or cow once grown.

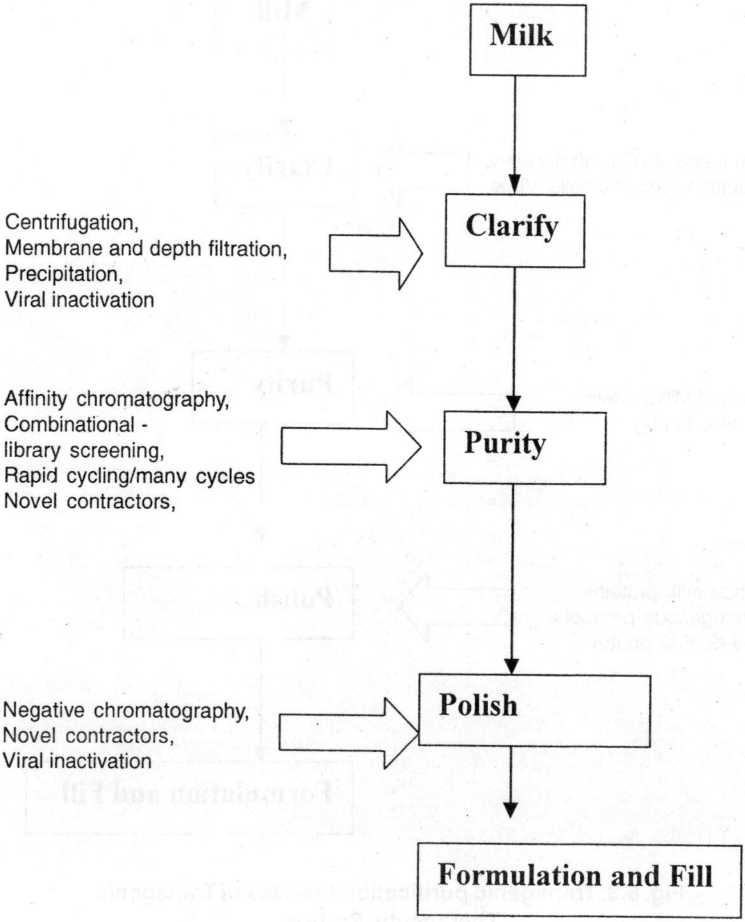

Fig. 6.2: Key of the Purification Technology of Transgenic Therapeutic Protein.

This procedure was carried out successfully by American scientists and the results were published in 1994.1 The human gene they used codes for Protein C that acts to control blood clotting. They obtained one gram of Protein C from each liter of milk produced by the pig. This is 200 times the concentration found in human blood plasma. Only about one third of the Protein C obtained was

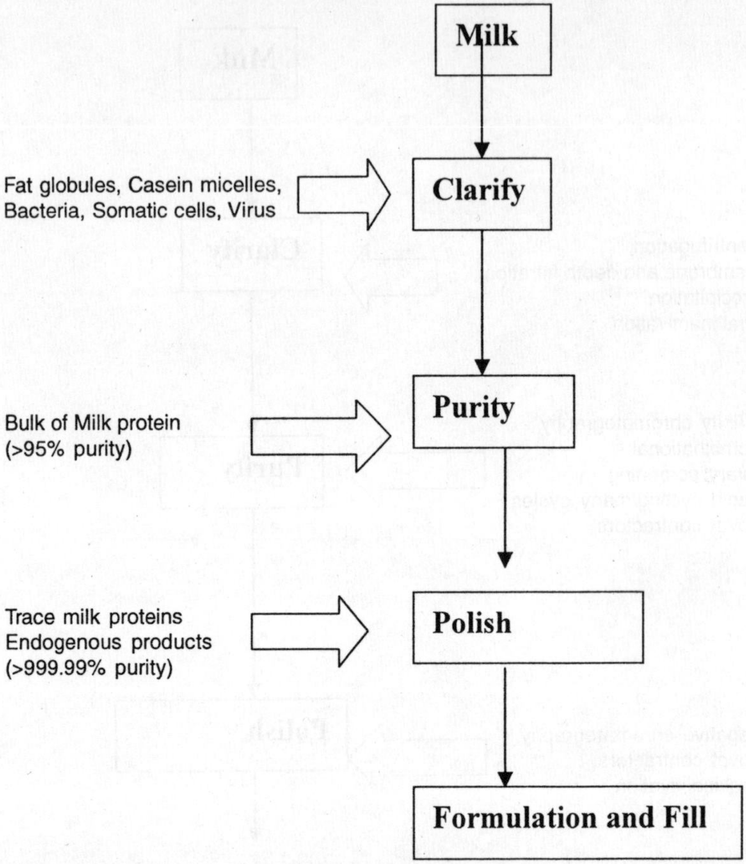

Fig. 6.3: Transgenic purification Process of Transgenic Therapeutic Protein.

biologically active. The reason for this is that many modifications of a protein must be performed in a cell after the protein chain is formed. For example, sections are cut out of the protein; complex sugar groups may be attached at certain places in the protein chain; and cell wall anchor groups may be added. The scientists discovered that a key processing enzyme, called furin, was present in insufficient quantities, so they added to their gene complex the gene that codes for furin. This increased the yield of active Protein C. The human proteins produced in this way must be tested for safety and effectiveness. Now, an anti-clotting protein called anti-thrombin is now being tested in clinical trials.

Comparing this procedure to the use of bioreactor machines illustrates the fact that a generation of biochemical engineers failed to match the abilities of a tool for making proteins (the pig or cow) that God had prepared. The mammary gland is optimized to maintain a high density of cells to deliver to them an ample supply of nutrients and to channel proteins that are produced in a form that can easily be isolated and purified. This procedure has proven to be successful and promises to provide a method for producing valuable therapeutic proteins at much lower cost.

Chapter 7
Synthetic Peptide

Peptides and Their Discovery

Every now and then a new discovery considerably widens the horizon of possible benefit to humankind. Someone theorized in 1980 that increased blood volume in some patients with heart disease or high blood pressure might stretch the weakest component in the vascular system and the body might register a protest in the blood. Such a weak spot is the entrance hall (called an atrium in Greek) to the heart pumps (ventricles). This led to intravenous injection of an extract of rat atrial tissue in rats. A copious natriuresis, or loss of sodium and water, resulted. (Natrium for sodium and oesis for water making.) So the first member of a family of peptides was found.

Peptides are chains of amino acids. As well as these effects the peptides relaxed blood vessels and protected the body against raised blood pressure and increased blood volume.

Types of Peptides

Three types of peptides share 17 amino acids with different head and tail amino acids attached.

They are atrial natriuretic peptide (ANP), brain natriuretic peptide (BNP), and C-type natriuretic peptide (CNP) under varying hormone or neurotransmitter control.

How Peptide Works in Our Body

Their effect varies according to where there is a docking (receptor) site. They then trigger cGMP controlled signals. Their action ends when endopeptidases (aminoacid clippers) in the kidney or blood vessels inactivate them. Some act directly on the brain to decrease salt appetite and water drinking. They also subdue signals from the sympathetic nervous system and inhibit deleterious overgrowth of damaged heart muscle. Similar peptides in the gastrointestinal tract regulate salt and water transport across the gut wall.

The natriuretic peptides therefore defend the body against excess salt and water retention. Patients with congestive heart failure, that is swollen edematous legs and severe shortness of breath, have high circulating levels of ANP and BNP; as much as 30 times normal. These high levels predispose them to abnormal heart rhythms and a poor survival outlook. Later in severe failure the levels fall as the circulation in the kidney fails. Something similar happens in the blood volume overload of kidney failure.

Drug Discovery and Peptides

A significant and growing portion of new drug discovery and development is being focused on a class of biomolecules called peptides. Peptides are polymers of amino acids that have biological functions determined by the exact arrangement, or sequence, of different amino acids in their makeup. There are 21 naturally occurring amino acids that in various combinations and permutations, make up the peptides and proteins of living things. Virtually every life process involves peptides in some way.

As the human genome project unfolds, thousands of different peptides and proteins with unique biological functions are being identified. As might be expected, many disease states are found to be influenced by these peptides and proteins. Accordingly, peptide based drug candidates are being discovered at an increasingly rapid pace, and a variety of new peptide drugs are being developed as therapeutics for cancers, pain management, viral infections, diabetes, and a host of endocrine and neurological disorders.

Some Important Synthetic Peptides

Salmon Calcitonin

Indications

Used for Osteoporosis

Available as nasal spray and injections.

Buserelin

Indications

It is indicated for the treatment of cancer of the prostate gland.

Available as nasal solution and injections.

Carbetocin

Indications

It is indicated for the treatment of control bleeding after delivery.

Available as nasal solution, nasal spray and injections.

Desmopression

Indications

1. Used to control the frequent urination, increased thirst and loss of water associated with diabetes insipidus.
2. Used to control the frequent urination, increased thirst and loss of water associated with certain types of brain injuries and brain surgery.
3. Desmopression is also given by injection to treat some patients with certain breeding problem such as hemophilia or von Willebrand's disease.

Goserelin

Indications

1. Cancer of the prostate
2. Cancer of the breast in woman if it develops before or around the time of menopause
3. Endometriosis, apainful condition caused by extra tissue growing inside or outside of the uterus
4. Thinning of the lining of the uterus before surgery on the uterus

Available as injection.

Gonadorelin

Indications

Used to cause ovulation (release of an egg from the ovary) in women who do not have regular ovulation and menstrual periods.

Available as injection.

Somatotasin

Indications

1. Several acute hemorrhages from esophageal region, gastric or duodenal ulcer or acute eorosive or hemorrhagic gastritis.
2. Complications following pancreatic sugery

Available as injection

Astracurium Besylate

Indications

For muscle relaxation in surgical anesthesia.

Available as injection

Triptorelin

Indications

Triptorelin decreases testosterone levels. Reducing the amount of testosterone in the body is one way to treat the prostate cancer.

Available as injection.

Peptide Synthesis

Chemically linking amino acids together to make a polypeptide chain.

Peptide Bond

The covalent linkage between the α-carboxyl end of one amino acid with the α-amino end of a second amino acid.

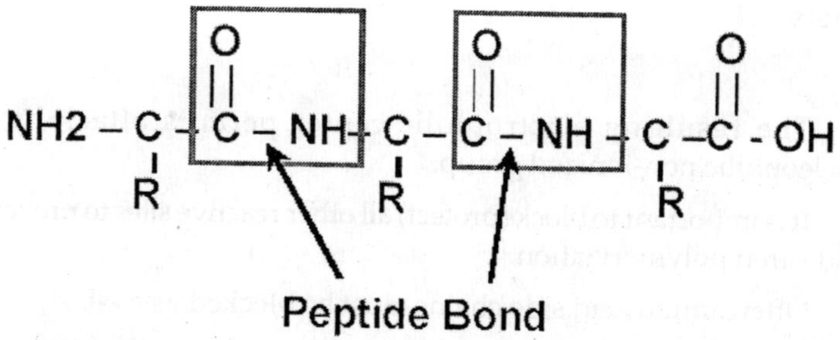

Fig. 7.1: Example of Peptide bonds

- Peptide Bond formation does not occur spontaneously. Requires activation of one of the two end groups, usually the carboxyl end.
- Increase the electrophilic character (reactivity) of the carbon atom buy pulling electron density away from it by adding a covalently linked activating substituent.

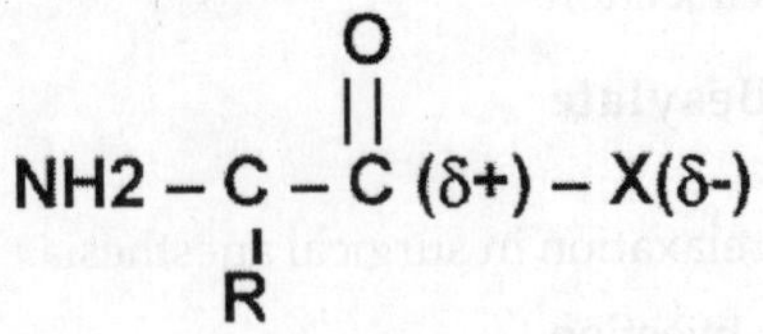

Fig. 7.2: Example of increase the electrophilic character

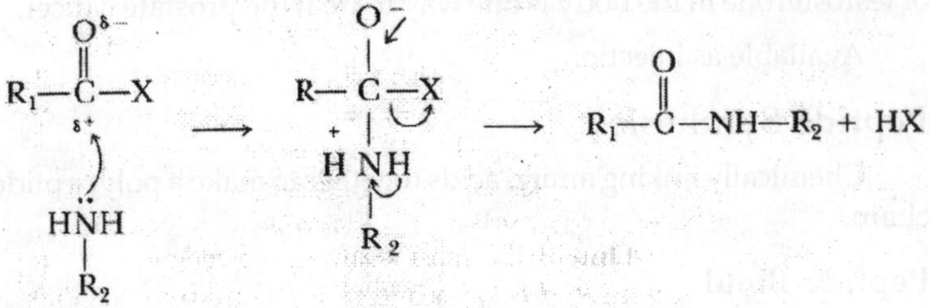

Fig. 7.3: Electrophilic center permits attack by a nucleophilic non-ionized group (X= azides, acid chlorides, mixed anhydrides, activated esters)

The resulting electrophilic center permits attack by a nucleophilic non-ionized group.

It is important to block (protect) all other reactive sites to prevent undesired polymerization.

Often amino acid side chains must be blocked as well.

It is important to use different protecting groups on the different parts of the amino acid to be able to selectively remove only one type of protecting group at a time.

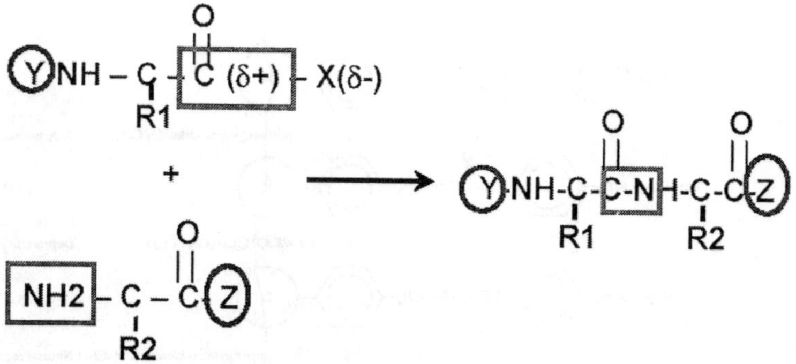

Fig. 7.4: To continue the polymerization above with addition of R3, you need to remove Z and replace it with X, without changing Y

Example of Solid Phase Synthesis of a 4 amino acid long peptide chain G-E-S-G

The efficiency of each cycle is critical for the success of a given synthesis. If complete deprotection or coupling causes a fraction of the new peptides to have the incorrect sequence. This is a cumulative effect.

Example: If the efficiency of adding each successive amino acid to a chain is 90% (which is pretty good in chemical synthesis):

After 10 amino acids only 35% of the chains would have the correct sequence.

After 20 amino acids only 12% would be correct

After 100 amino acids only 0.003% would be correct

Even with extreme accuracy (99% efficiency) on 37 % of chains would be correct after 100 amino acids.

If you want to make a long protein, you are better off to synthesis and purify smaller fragments and then join them together.

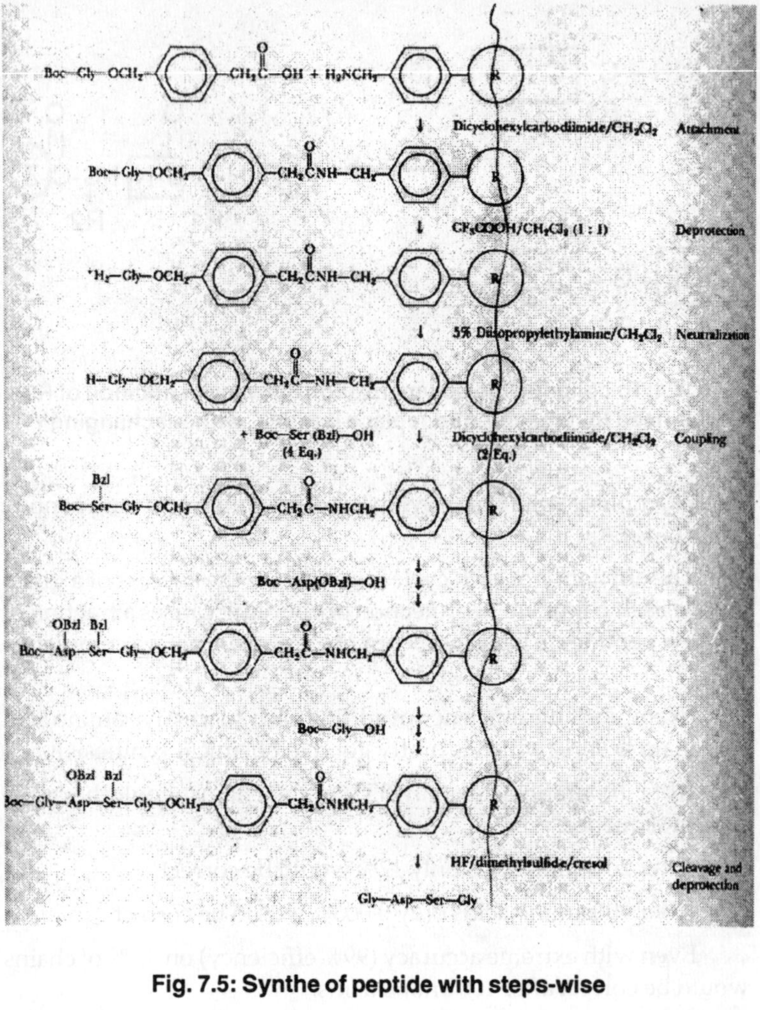

Fig. 7.5: Synthe of peptide with steps-wise

Chapter 8

Drug Delivery and Formulation

In recent years, the number of protein-based pharmaceuticals reaching the marketplace has increased exponentially. The clinical application of these drugs is limited by a lack of desirable attributes for adequate absorption or distribution. It therefore becomes critical to formulate these drugs into safe, stable and efficacious delivery systems. Most protein products currently on the market are for parenteral administration; however, half-lives are short and they would benefit from the development of controlled release parenterals. Among non-invasive delivery methods, one of the most promising approaches is pulmonary delivery. The following discussion pertains mostly to these two approaches, i.e. controlled parenteral or pulmonary delivery; however, significant and successful work is also being undertaken to deliver proteins by oral, transdermal, nasal and other mucosal routes. Approaches being investigated for oral delivery of proteins include the use of site-specific delivery to sites within the gastrointestinal tract that have less proteolytic activity, and the use of protease inhibitors, bioadhesive delivery systems, penetration enhancers, carrier systems or formulation approaches. Many of these approaches are being used in conjunction with proprietary technologies such as the carrier systems being used by Emisphere Technologies for oral delivery of macromolecules such as heparin, calcitonin and insulin. Modified drug forms such as the hexyl insulin-amphiphilic polymer conjugate from Nobex

Corporation are also being investigated in clinical studies for oral delivery. Similarly, nasal delivery is being investigated. The cells of the nasal mucosa overlay a rich vasculature from which drugs can be absorbed readily for a fast onset of action. Several small peptides, as well as a larger polypeptide, calcitonin, are available commercially for nasal delivery.

Parenteral Delivery

Currently, peptide and protein drugs are marketed almost exclusively for parenteral administration. This is because these drugs face formidable enzymatic and penetration barriers when administered orally. A limitation of the parenteral route for delivery of peptides and proteins is the extremely short half-lives of these drugs - in the order of a few minutes. This demands repeated administration, which is inconvenient to the patient. For this reason, nonparenteral routes of administration are being investigated actively. Another alternative is to develop controlled release parenteral formulations, where a single injection may release the drug over a month or even longer. Some of the most promising approaches include PEGylation and microspheres. Other methods to develop controlled release parenteral delivery systems include oil-based injections, implants, liposomes, nanoparticles and pumps. Solid lipid nanoparticles are also being developed as alternative carrier systems to traditional colloidal carriers such as liposomes and polymeric particles. Lipids that are well tolerated by the body are used to coat the drug particles. Large-scale production is feasible in a cost-effective manner. Drug delivery systems with a pulsatile release pattern are being developed for drugs where prolonged continuous release is not desired, for example for drugs that have special chronopharmacological needs. Implants that can be inserted directly into the affected area during surgery will also play an important role in drug delivery systems. Needle-free injections that work by forcing medication at high speed through the skin are already on the market. These work by creating a fine stream of high-pressure fluid to penetrate the skin and deposit the drug in the underlying tissue.

PEGylation

Conjugation of proteins to polyethylene glycol (PEG) is perhaps the most common approach to chemical modification of a protein for several potential beneficial effects. These can include increased bioavailability, increased plasma half-lives, decreased immunogenicity, reduced proteolysis and enhanced solubility and stability. Several PEG-protein products are currently under development. Products that have been on the market for some time include PEG-adenosine deaminase (Adagen® - Enzon/NPS Pharmaceuticals) and PEG-asparaginase (Oncaspar® - Rhone-Poulenc Rorer). More recently, PEG-interferon as peginterferon alfa-2b (PEG-INTRON® - Schering- Plough) and Peginterferon alfa-2a (PEGASYS® - Roche) were approved by the US Food and Drug Administration (FDA) for treatment of chronic hepatitis C by parenteral administration. Due to an increase in size of the interferon molecule, pegylated interferon has a slower absorption rate, prolonged half-life and reduced clearance. It therefore needs less frequent administration. Tolerability of the pegylated interferons is comparable with the non-pegylated formulations. Several more products are under investigation. The two interferons, as well as pegfilgrastim (Neulasta® - Amgen) and pegvisomant (Somavert® - Pharmacia), use the PEGylation technology of Nektar Therapeutics, which was formed by the merger of Inhale Therapeutics, Shearwater Corporation and Bradford Particle Design. STEALTH® liposomes (Alza Corporation) have also been designed by PEG coating to enable them to escape recognition by the immune system.

Microspheres

Microspheres are free-flowing powders, ideally less than about 125μm in diameter, which can be suspended in suitable aqueous vehicles for injection with a conventional syringe using an 18 or 20-gauge needle. The most promising polymers for such use are lactide/glycolide co-polymers, poly(ortho esters) and polyanhydrides. Poly (D,L-lactide-co-glycolide) (PLGA) is a biodegradable polymer that hydrolyses with an acid or base-catalysed reaction to form the natural metabolites glycolic and lactic acid. PLGA is FDA-approved. Currently, there is one microsphere peptide formulation on the US market. This formulation contains a synthetic analogue of luteinising hormone-releasing hormone leuprolide acetate (Lupron Depot®). Microencapsulation of proteins into microspheres may have more limitation compared with peptides. This is because proteins have a more complex structure, characterised by a well-defined tertiary structure that may be affected by the harsh manufacturing conditions of the conventional emulsification process used for microsphere preparation. More recently, microspheres of a therapeutic protein, recombinant human growth hormone (rhGH) Nutropin Depot® - Genentech, Inc.), were produced using a ProLease® technology (Alkermes, Inc.). In the ProLease® process, a different approach is used. A lyophilised protein powder is dispersed in a polymer solution and atomised into liquid nitrogen. The solvent is then extracted from frozen microspheres. An aseptic process can be used where solutions are filtered using 0.22μm filters into an isolator, and pre-sterilised solid components are introduced into the isolator aseptically using rapid transfer ports. All the production steps occur in the isolator to result in a sterile product. This process is feasible at a commercially viable scale under current Good Manufacturing Practice (GMP) conditions (30).

Formulation Approach

A formulation approach to protein delivery is also being pursued actively. Non-aqueous formulations for recombinant proteins such as leuprolide acetate, rhGH, glucagon-like peptide-1 (GLP-1), recombinant human interferon gamma (rhu-IFN) and recombinant human relaxin have been reported to be stable for three months to more than one year at 37°C. Leuprolide formulated in dimethyl sulphoxide is on the market as Viadur a once-yearly implant for the palliative treatment of advanced prostate cancer. This product uses Alza's DUROS implant technology and provides continuous, 12-month suppression of testosterone with single treatment.

A SABER delivery system from Southern BioSystems is also under development. This is a biodegradable gel that consists of sucrose acetate isobutyrate (SAIB), a solvent and a polymeric release modifier. SAIB is a very hydrophobic, fully esterified sucrose derivative that exists as a very viscous liquid and is approved as a food additive in many countries. Upon injection, the solvent diffuses away from the SAIB and the viscosity increases dramatically to provide sustained release of the protein incorporated into the gel/ viscous depot.

In addition, recent advances in our understanding of macromolecular crystallisation are making it possible to crystallise proteins.

Companies such as Altus Biologics have scaled up the process and crystallised monoclonal antibodies, and have shown that the resulting product is stable and bioactive.

Formulation for Lyophilized Protein Parenteral

For lyophilized parenteral preparations, as with any dosage form, product design parameters and objectives define the focus and direct the efforts in product development. Design parameters need to consider pharmacological, clinical and physio-chemical aspects of the active ingredient. These encompass the therapeutic response, administration, and stability requirements.

The therapeutic response entails the therapeutic regime and route administration. A regime may range from a single injection to multiple routine administrations. Single administration may be for an acute condition or vaccination. Short-term administration of oncology preparations for chemotherapy is often intermittent. IV therapy of antibiotics is used as a post-operative prophylactic. Long-term therapy may require relatively frequent administration, as in anti-hemophilia therapy.

Routes of administration also vary. The three most common routes are intravenous, intramuscular, and subcutaneous. Some less common routes are intraocular, intrathecal, intra-arterial, and intra-articular. Volumes of an injection, influenced by solubility of the active ingredient, need to take into account the preferred route of administration. A therapy may require a bolus injection of 10 ml in 10 minutes, an intermittent infusion of 50 or 100 ml using a "piggyback" i.v. administration system, or a continuous infusion over several hours or days . Intramuscular injections of 2 ml are not uncommon. Smaller volumes of 0.5 to 1.5 ml are appropriate for subcutaneous injection.

Factors necessary in achieving adequate finished product characteristics include physio-chemical, microbiological, therapeutic and toxicological aspects. Lyophilization is principally a method of preservation for products that degrade in solution due to reactions with water. Products may also be light and oxygen sensitive. Providing adequate stability is a major product and process design objective for a lyophilized therapeutic. Sufficient stability is necessary to allow for preparation and processing during manufacturing that includes bulk solution preparation, sterile filtration, filling, and loading into the lyophilizer. Stability of the constituted solution is also important for convenient clinical use. The product design, focusing on the product formulation, also needs to provide sufficient stability in the dried state to accommodate adequate time for distribution and storage until final use.

Loss of potency may be attributable to direct chemical degradation or structural alteration. Chemical reactions readily occur in solution and can also occur in the dried state. These reactions include hydrolysis, oxidation, isomerization, and deamidation. Structural alteration of peptides and proteins is mostly but not exclusively associated with biopharmaceuticals. These alterations may manifest as precipitation, adsorption onto the glass vial, reversible and irreversible denaturation, polymerization and aggregation .

The objective for any lyophilized preparation is stability through the expiry date to provide sufficient chemical/biochemical recovery upon reconstitution in order to achieve the desired therapeutic effect. This also assumes the absence of any significant amount of degradation products. Parenteral products, regardless of the administration routes must meet all the criteria for an injection defined in the USP . They need to be no less clear than the diluent, be completely in solution, with no visible residue of undissolved material, and essentially free of visible particulate matter. These preparations must also be sterile and with a sufficiently low level of endotoxin.

Factors in Formulation Design

The formulation consists of the active ingredient and may include excipients with various functions. Formulation design needs to take into account the active pharmaceutical ingredient (API), and specific function and effects of excipients, concentration of the active and the excipients, isotonicity, and pH (28).

The formulation design and choice of excipients need to take into consideration the requirements of the API, route, volume and frequency of administration, influence on stability, and requirements for processing . Excipients used for lyophile preparations may be categorized into their principle functions.

Following figure highlights these classes and provides examples of each.

Fig. 8.1: Highlights Different Classes of Excipients for Formulation Design of Protein Drugs

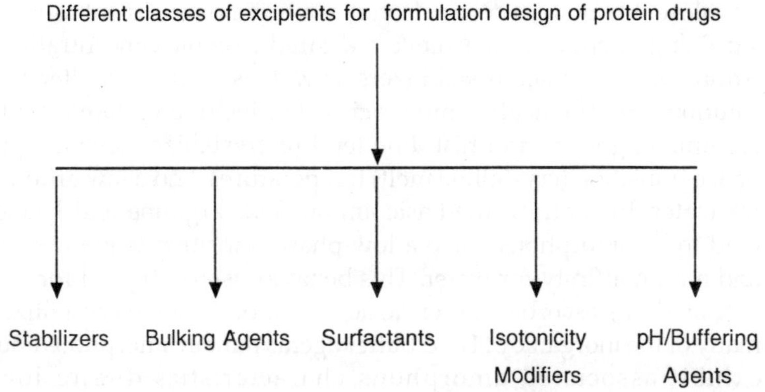

Excipients often have a predominant use and advantage in a formulation. Examples of common excipients used in lyophilized products categorized according to their prominent characteristics are presented in Table 8.1. It is important to note that some excipients may be used to achieve multiple effects in a formulation. For example, mannitol may be used as a bulking agent and to achieve a desired isotonic concentration for the reconstituted solution. Surfactants are present with peptides and proteins to minimize intermolecular adsorption and aggregation. Citric acid / sodium citrate may be used for pH adjustment, as a chelating agent and anti-oxidant.

Table 8.1: Commonly Used Excipients and their Categories

Stabilizers Bulking Agents	*Acidic Amino Acids*	*Basic Amino Acids*	*Organic Acids/ Acids*	*Surfac- tants Bases*	*Inor- ganic Acids*	*Inor- ganic Bases*	*Inor- ganic Salts*
Lacose	Glutamine	Arginine	Acetic	Tween	HCl	NaOH	KCl
Maltose	Glycine	Lysine	Acid/ Acetate	Pluronic	Phosphoric	Dibasic	NaCl
Mannitol	Histidine		Amino Acids			Phosphate	
Sucrose	Leucine		Citric/Citrate				
Trehalose	Threonine		Ascorbic Ascorbate				

Many excipients exhibit characteristic behaviors when frozen and freeze dried as simple aqueous preparations. Saccharides used as both stabilizers and bulking agents tend to be amorphous, have low phase transition (collapse) temperatures and a high affinity for water. Common saccharides include lactose, maltose, sucrose and trehalose. Mannitol, a sugar alcohol, is a common excipient used as a bulking agent and to achieve a desired isotonic concentration. Amino acids can act as stabilizers as well as be used to alter the solution pH. The acidic amino acids that include glutamic acid, glutamine, glycine and histidine tend to crystallize, have a high phase transition (crystalline melt) temperatures, and a low affinity for water. In contrast, the basic amino acids arginine and lysine tend to be amorphous, have a low phase transition temperature, and a high affinity for water. This behavior is also typical for the anti-oxidants ascorbic and citric acid. Although some crystallize, many of the inorganic pH and buffer agents remain amorphous and exhibit associated amorphous characteristics due to low concentrations used and effects of other excipients.

Behavior of an excipient would be expected to be different when in the presence of an API or when different excipients are combined. It is desirable to design a formulation using the simplest combination of excipients with a specific function for each. Some combinations of excipients may have synergistic effects, and overall, the formulation will behave most like the principal constituent, depending upon the molar ratio. For example, an aqueous formulation containing a low concentration of a highly potent compound as an API and sucrose as both a stabilizer and bulking agent with a small amount of sodium chloride to adjust the isotonicity may behave similar to a simple sucrose solution. In contrast, when a small amount of citric acid is added to a mannitol formulation, the preparation behaves very differently than the mannitol alone. A mannitol and citric acid formulation with NaOH to adjust the pH, compared to combinations of mannitol, arginine and HCl and mannitol, glycine and NaOH will all behave differently. For example, processing times for these mannitol preparations in completing sublimation of ice during primary drying were 22 hours when containing citric acid, 36 hours when containing arginine and 38 hours when containing glycine .

Interaction of various excipients and their relative molar concentration are important to consider when designing the formulation. Their effect on behavior during processing, the conditions needed to successfully process the preparation, along with the effect of finished product attributes such as residual moisture also needs to be considered. For example, the mannitol formulations containing citric acid, arginine and glycine described above and processed using the same parameters yielded residual moistures of 3.9%, 0.1% and 0.4%, respectively .

Product Presentation and Processing Aspects

In addition to being influenced by the formulation, processing requirements must also take solution volume and container/closure used into account (29). For example, time to complete sublimation during primary drying for a 4 mL fill volume of a 7.5% w/v sucrose formulation in a 10 mL tubing vial has been measured as approximately 70 hours as compared to 25 hours for the same volume in a 20 mL tubing vial using the same shelf temperature and chamber pressure for lyophilization. Altering the concentration of the formulation can also have a significant effect.

Predicting the behavior of a presentation can include the use of the excipients alone or with slight modification as a model of the actual product presentation. For example, a model formulation containing mannitol, glycine and phosphate behaves like the actual product when the concentration of the API is low. In contrast, a sucrose, phosphate buffer and polysorbate formulation requires the substitution of human serum albumin to emulate the behavior of the formulation containing a relatively high concentration of a therapeutic protein: the formulation without the protein behaves significantly different. The need for such a substitution strongly depends on the formulation and nature of the API.

Selection of Process Parameters

The critical process parameters for lyophilization are shelf temperature, chamber pressure and time. Shelf temperature influences product temperature and has the greatest impact on rates during processing. Chamber pressure has the greatest effect on product temperature, and to a lesser degree, drying rates, due to the influence on heat transfer. There is a minimal time in order to fully complete solidification during freezing, sublimation during primary drying, and desorption to achieve a sufficiently low residual moisture during secondary drying.

The shelf temperature selected is dependent on both the formulation and product presentation. Influencing factors on behavior during processing derived from the formulation and product presentation include API and excipient characteristics, phase transition temperature, solute concentration, fill volume, vial size and vial type. A significant factor is the phase transition temperature. A collapse temperature associated with a phase transition such as -32 °C of a sucrose formulation requires low shelf temperatures and chamber pressures. These conservative processing conditions result in longer processing times. The low shelf temperature leads to slower processing rates. Chamber pressure, controlled to a portion of the pressure corresponding to the vapor pressure of ice at the product phase transition temperature, has long been acknowledged to be necessary for adequate process control . A low pressure would help maintain the product below the glass transition and avoid the opportunity for collapse. Product behavior also influences achievable processing rates and resulting time for completing each step, and is strongly influenced by factors including, fill volume, formulation, vial type and vial size.

Clearly defining the design parameters and objectives in developing a product and process prior to beginning development leads to successful results with less effort expended and reduced development time. Designing a product suitable for the therapy and route of administration are of the highest priority. Once product design criteria are satisfied, emphasis needs to be placed on promoting stability of the active ingredient in both solution and the dried state. From these design parameters comes the formulation and volume, and from the fill and final reconstitution volume, a minimum vial size. After designing a product presentation that meets these needs, attention can be given to processing conditions necessary for routine product manufacturing.

Although presented in a rational progression, therapeutic aspects, needs of the API, formulation characteristics, product presentation and processing are each interrelated such that critical requirements and desirable attributes need to be considered when designing a product. Designing a final presentation that takes influential product aspects into account allows for development of a manufacturing process that is effective and efficient. Design aspects also need to impart sufficient stability, appropriate attributes for administration to achieve the desired therapeutic effect, while providing a final product that is easily used in a clinical setting.

Some example of commonly Used excipients for proteins drugs are as follows

rhu EPO
Solution for injection

Ingredient	*Specification*	*Purpose of Use*
Erythropoietin	IHS	Erythropoiesis stimulating factor
Sodium chloride	USP XXIV	To produce isotonicity
Albumin human	USP XXIV	Stabilizing agent
Sodium phosphate dibasic dihydrate	USP XXIV	To produce buffer effect.
Sodium phosphate monobasic dihydrate	USP XXIV	To produce buffer effect.
Water for injection	USP XXIV	Solvent

IHS: In house specification

Each vial contains

EPO	2,000 UI
r-hu-erythropoietin	2,000 UI
Sodium chloride	5.80 mg
Sodium phosphate monobasic dihydrate	1.164 mg
Sodium phosphate dibasic dihydrate	2.225 mg
Albumin human	2.50 mg
Water for injection q.s.	1.00 ml

rhu G-CSF
Injectable Vials and pre-filled syringes

Ingredient	*Specification*	*Purpose of Use*
R-Met-hu-G-CSF	IHS	Stimulating Factor for the proliferation of Granulocyte cells
Glacial Acetic Acid	USP XXIV	To adjust the pH of final solution
Sodium Acetate	USP XXIV	Buffer
Mannitol	USP XXIV	Stabilizing agent
Polisorbate 80	USP XXIV	Stabilizing agent
Water for injections	USP XXIV	Solvent

Solution for Injection Vial 30 MIU

Ingredient		Specification	Quantity
R-Met-hu-G-CSF	⊗	IHS	300 μg
Glacial Acetic Acid		USP XXIV	0.50 mg
Sodium Acetate		USP XXIV	0.123 mg
Mannitol		USP XXIV	50.00 mg
Polisorbate 80		USP XXIV	0.04 mg
Water for injections q.s.		USP XXIV	1.00 ml

rhu GM-CSF

Ingredient		Specification	Quantity
R-hu-GM-CSF	⊗	IHS	300 μg
Mannitol		USP XXIV	50.00 mg
Sodium phosphate dibasic		USP XXIV	2.60 mg
Citric acid		USP XXIV	0.28 mg
Polyethylene glycol		USP XXIV	0.10 mg
Human Albumin		USP XXIV	1.00 mg

Ingredient	Specification	Purpose of Use
R-hu-GM-CSF	IHS	Active Ingredient
Mannitol	USP XXIV	Stabilizer
Sodium phosphate dibasic	USP XXIV	To adjust the pH of final solution
Citric acid	USP XXIV	To adjust the pH of final solution
Polyethylene glycol	USP XXIV	Stabilizer
Human Albumin	USP XXIV	Stabilizer

rhu Interferon (IFN) alpha-2b

Ingredient		Specification	Quantity
Interferon alpha-2b	⊗	IHS	15 μg
Glycine		USP XXIV	20.00 mg
Albumin human		USP XXIV	1.00 mg
Sodium phosphate dibasic		USP XXIV	2.27 mg
Sodium phosphate monobasic monohydrate		USP XXIV	0.55 mg
Water for injection (to dilut.)		USP XXIV	1.00 ml

Ingredient	*Specification*	*Purpose of Use*
Interferon (IFN) alpha-2b	IHS	Immunomodulator, antineoplastic
Glycine	USP XXIV	Acidifying agent
Albumin human	USP XXIV	Stabilizer agent essential for preservation of the active ingredient during lyophilization.
Sodium phosphate dibasic	USP XXIV	To produce buffer effect.
Sodium phosphate monobasic monohydrate	USP XXIV	To produce buffer effect.

INF dilution vial

Ingredient	*Specification*	*Purpose of Use*
Water for injection	USP XXIV	solvent

Chapter 9

World Scenario

During the past two decades, the medical biotechnology industry has successfully brought more than 160 drugs and vaccines to the marketplace. Additionally, according to the Pharmaceutical Research and Manufacturing Association (PHRMA), there are over 371 new products currently in clinical trials targeting more than 200 diseases. These include AIDS, Alzheimer's disease, arthritis, cancer, diabetes, heart disease, and multiple sclerosis. A large proportion of these drugs are protein-based therapeutics, which are primarily injectables and are generally more expensive than small-molecule drugs. Indeed, a year's supply of some of the protein drugs could be in the range of $10,000 or more. For example, recently approved Rebif®, a form of interferon β-1a for the treatment of relapsing forms of multiple sclerosis, is available in the U.S., and according to Serono (Geneva, Switzerland), the maker of the drug, it will cost the patient $1445 per month ($17,344 per year). In spite of the expense for some of the disease treatments, the use of protein therapeutics is the only option a patient has. This application note highlights a few of the salient statistics of biomedicines and the future challenges and prospects they face.

Revenue Growth

Since the FDA's approval in 1982 of recombinant insulin as the first recombinant biopharmaceutical, many biotechnology companies and traditional pharmaceutical companies have devoted their resources to discover and develop numerous recombinant protein medicines. As a result, currently about 80 drugs, or 50% of the total approved biotechnology drugs, are protein therapeutics. Some of the biomedicines, as shown in Table 9.1, are already blockbuster products that generate more than half a billion to multibillion dollars per drug in annual revenue. Overall, biotechnology drugs make up only a small percentage, approximately 8% of the total annual revenues generated by the pharmaceutical industry. The worldwide pharmaceutical market brought in $364 billion in 2001 sales (Table 9.2), of which $28.5 billion was generated from biotechnology products. This was a more than 500% increase over that of 1989, which saw $4.7 billion revenues (source: Biotechnology Industry Organization, Washington, DC). Interestingly, five of the pioneering biotechnology companies- Amgen, Genentech, Chiron (Emeryville, CA),

Genzyme, and Biogen-generated one-third of the 2001 revenue, $9.39 billion, primarily through the sale of their biomedicines. Several pharmaceutical companies, such as Johnson & Johnson, Eli Lilly, Roche, Bayer (Berkeley, CA), and Schering Plough, remain at the forefront of the biotherapeutics revolution primarily through their acquisition of products for further development or by becoming marketing partners of various smaller to medium-size biotechnology companies. In fact, in most of the cases, this has been a valuable and productive strategy, since some of the highest revenue generating biomedicines are the products of such joint ventures demonstrated in Figure 9.1. Starting with a mere $9 million revenue in 1980, the companies collected 12 billion in 2002, a spectacular growth indeed. Even during the difficult financial period of the last three years, revenue rose to an average of about 25% annually. Each of these companies has multiple biomedicines on the market, as well as in their developmental pipeline. For example, Amgen is the larget biotherapeutics company, with a 2002 revenue of $5.5 billion, an increase of 38% over that of 2001, generated by the sale of several of its breakthrough biotherapeutics such as Aranesp, Enbrel, Epogen, Kineret, Neulasta, and Neupogen. Currently, the company has seven products in various stages of development.

Genentech, the second largest in the group, generated $2.7 billion in 2002, an increase of 24% over its 2001 sales. Its marketed biomedicines include Herceptin and Rituxan for oncology treatment, Activase and TNKase as vascular medicine, the growth hormone

Neutropin as a metabolic drug, and Pulmozyme for the treatment of cystic fibrosis patients. The company's antibody drug, Xolair, was recently approved. Additionally, it has at least a half dozen monoclonal antibodies in various stages of development.

Chiron reported 2002 total revenues of $1.3 billion, which amounted to an 18% increase in product sales over 2001. Of this, the net product sales and royalty income of the company's biopharmaceutical division amounted to $456 million.

Chiron's product pipeline includes several combination drugs involving monoclonal antibodies, such as Proleukin aldesleukin) interleukin-2 + rituximab refractory for low-grade non- Hodgkin's lymphoma (NHL), Proleukin + rituximab + chemotherapy refractory for high-grade NHL, liquid IL-2/rituximab for NHL, and liquid IL-2/trastuzumab for breast cancer.

Genzyme generated revenue of $1.33 billion, primarily from sales of Cerezyme, up about 9% compared to 1.224 million for the previous year. recently obtained approval for Fab- razyme and Aldurazyme, treatments for lysosomal storage disorders it developed in collaboration with BioMarin Pharmaceutical of Novato, CA. It has several protein drugs, including monoclonal antibodies, in development. Biogen's revenue in 2002 increased by 10% over that of 2001, to $1.14 billion from the sale of five marketed products: Amevive® (alefacept), Avonex (interferon β-1a), Intron® A (interferon α-2b, recombinant), Energix-B®/Recombivax® (hepatitis B vaccines), and Angiomax® (bivalirudin). While it has several biotherapeutics in its developmental pipeline, it recently announced a merger with IDEC Pharmaceuticals, the San Diego, Cabased antibody company. The combined revenue of the two companies for 2002 was $1.55 billion, making it the third largest biotechnology company (34).

Prospects

It is generally believed that most of the naturally occurring, well-studied proteins that have therapeutic potential have already been discovered. Consequently, the threshold for discovering protein drugs with unique biological efficacy has increased substantially. The current approach is to utilize the genomics and proteomics technologies and discover otherwise more difficult-to-find proteins of therapeutic importance, or generate the socalled designer proteins that can be utilized as therapeutics. Despite such stringency, many companies are involved in the protein drug business since the payoff from discovering a good protein drug is enormous. As demonstrated in Table 9.1, many of the current protein drugs are indeed blockbusters, earning more than half to a multibillion dollar annual revenues. Additionally, a recombinant protein offers an exclusive intellectual property position to a company. Since most protein therapeutics provide a positive effect in a biological phenomenon in contrast to an inhibitory function of most of the small-molecule drugs, less time in a clinical setting is required to determine the efficacy of the protein molecule. While the majority of the proteins are injectables, significant progress has been made in recent years to generate alternative delivery pathways such as oral or inhalation or self injectables, potentially alleviating cumbersome and expensive hospital stays or visits to clinics. In terms of oral delivery, which is currently the most promising, there are at least four sets of hurdles, both at the biological and economic fronts, cited by Emisphere Technology (Tarrytown, NY), one of the forerunners among over 300 drug delivery companies, according to a report from the market research firm, Frost and Sullivan. At the biological front, the primary challenge is to inhibit or slow down the degradation of protein drugs by the digestive tract enzymes before they are absorbed into the bloodstream. Additionally, the impact of dosing variability on efficacy needs to be overcome. At the economic front, attention needs to be paid to decreasing the production cost of the protein drugs. Indeed, in recent years, with the availability of various low-cost, high-volume production systems, many companies have begun working to generate products that are less expensive, and develop delivery efficiencies to create products with high profit margins. Only a few biotechnology companies have dominated the protein therapeutics industry for the past 27 years of the modern biotechnology industry. Not surprisingly, the market valuation of these companies has increased significantly as they successfully introduced products to the market. However, due to the increased competitive pressure and the shareholders' desire to cash in substantial value, some of these companies have subsequently fallen pray to acquisition cum consolidation. In some cases, such consolidation has taken place within the peergroup companies, while in others, larger pharmaceutical companies have become the acquirer. For example, Amgen acquired Immunex in 2002, and Biogen and IDEC recently

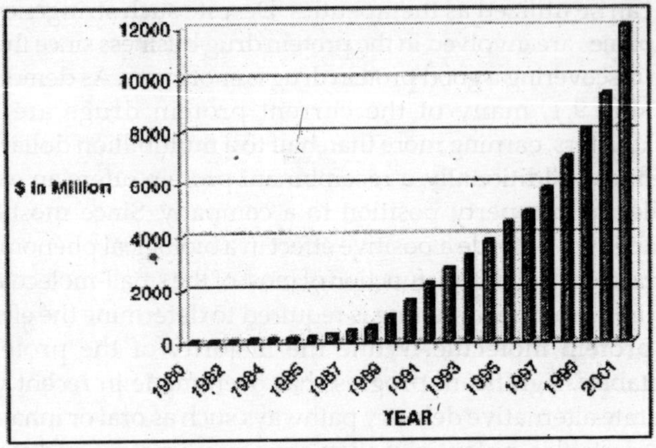

Fig. 9.1: Cumulative Revenues of Selected Biotechnology Companies. Data collected from BIO Web site (www.bio.org) and the annual reports of Amgen, Genentech, Chiron, Genzyme, and Biogen.

Table 9.1: Selected Blockbuster Protein Therapeutics

Product name	Constituent protein	Therapeutic impact/disease indication	Year of approval	Company (developer/ marketer)[b]	Worldwide sales, 2002 (in $ million)	Worldwide sales, 2001 (in $ million)	Percent increase or decrease
Avonex®	Interferon β-1a	Multiple sclerosis	1996	Biogen	1034	972	6.38
Betaseron®/betaferon	Interferon β-1b	Multiple sclerosis	1993	Schering AG	830	592	40.2
Cerezyme®/ceredase	Glucocerebrosidase	Gaucher disease	1991	Genzyme	619	570	8.6
Enbrel®	Etanercept (fusion protein of antibody-Fc and p75-TNF receptor protein)	Rheumatoid arthritis	1998	Immunex (presently Amgen)	802	762	5.2
Epogen®	Erythropoeitin	Stimulation of erythrocyte production	1989	Amgen	2300	2200	0.24
Herceptin®	Trastuzumab (anti-HER-2 antibody)	Breast cancer	1998	Genentech/Roche	715	537	33.15
Humalog®	Insulin	Diabetes	1996	Eli Lilly	834	628	32.8
Humulin®	Insulin	Diabetes	1982	Eli Lilly	1004	1061	(1.76)[c]
Intron®-A and Robetron®	α-Interferon and PEGylated α-interferon	Antitumor (anti-HIV)	1986 and 1998	Schering Plough	2700	1447	86.6
NeoRecormon®	Erythropoeitin β	Stimulation of erythrocyte production	1997 and 2002	Roche	1192	443	169
Neupogen®	G-CSF	Stimulation of granulocyte production	1991	Amgen	1400	1300	7.69
Procrit™/Eprex™	Erythropoeitin α	Stimulation of erythrocyte production	1993	Johnson & Johnson/Ortho Biotech	4283	3430	24.87
Rebif	Interferon β-1a	Multiple sclerosis	2002 (1998 in Europe)	Ares-Serono	549	380	44.47
Rituxan®	Rituximab (humanized antibody)	Leukemia and lymphomas	1997	Genentech/Roche	1650	1113	48.25
Remicade®	Infliximab (chimeric MAb)	Rheumatoid arthritis	1998	Centocor/Johnson & Johnson/Schering Plough	1146[d]	847	35.3
Synagis®	Humanized MAb	Respiratory syncytial virus prevention	1998	MedImmune/Abbott	668	516	29.46

Table 9.2: 2001 Global Pharmaceutical Sales

World audited market	2001 sales ($ billion)	% Growth (constant $)
North America	181.8	+17
Europe	88.0	+10
Japan	47.6	+4
Asia, Africa, and Australia	27.9	+9
Latin America	18.9	+0.1
Total	$364.2	+12

announced their merger. Genetics Institute has been acquired by Wyeth (Madison, NJ), and Centocor was bought by Johnson & Johnson. With the increassuccess of the biotherapeutics business, such consolidation trend should continue.

Chapter 10

Regulatory Aspects

It is important to keep in mind the realities of the drug discovery and development process. The U.S. system of new drug approvals is perhaps the most rigorous in the world. On average, it costs a company $359 million to get one new medicine from the laboratory to the pharmacist's shelf, according to a February 1993 report by the Congressional Office of Technology Assessment. It takes 12 years on average for an experimental drug to travel from lab to medicine chest. Only five in 5,000 compounds that enter preclinical testing make it to human testing. One of these five tested in people is approved. New medicines are developed as follows:

Synthesis and Extraction

The process of identifying new molecules with the potential to produce a desired change in a biological system (e.g., to inhibit or stimulate an important enzyme, to alter a metabolic pathway,or to change cellular structure). The process may require: 1) research on the fundamental mechanisms of disease or biological processes; 2) research on the action of known therapeutic agents; or 3) random selection and broad biological screening. New molecules can be produced through artificial synthesis or extracted from natural sources (plant, mineral, or animal). The number of compounds that can be produced based on the same general chemical structure runs into the hundreds of millions.

Biological Screening and Pharmacological Testing

Studies to explore the pharmacological activity and therapeutic potential of compounds. These tests involve the use of animals, isolated cell cultures and tissues, enzymes and cloned receptor sites as well as computer models. If the results of the tests suggest potential beneficial activity, related compounds Ñeach a unique structural modification of the originalÑ are tested to see which version of the molecule produces the highest level of pharmacological activity and demonstrates the most therapeutic promise, with the smallest number of potentially harmful biological properties.

Pharmaceutical Dosage Formulation and Stability Testing

The process of turning an active compound into a form and strength suitable for human use. A pharmaceutical product can take any one of a number of dosage forms (*e.g.*, liquid, tablets, capsules, ointments, sprays, patches) and dosage strengths (*e.g.*, 50. 100, 250, 500 mg.) The final formulation will include substances other than the active ingredient, called excipients. Excipients are added to improve the taste of an oral product, to allow the active ingredient to be compounded into stable tablets, to delay the drug's absorption into the body, or to prevent bacterial growth in liquid or cream preparations. The impact of each on the human body must be tested.

Toxicology and Safety Testing

Tests to determine the potential risk a compound poses to man and the environment. These studies involve the use of animals, tissue cultures, and other test systems to examine the relationship between factors such as dose level, frequency of administration, and duration of exposure to both the short- and long-term survival of living organisms. Tests provide information on the dose-response pattern of the compound and its toxic effects. Most toxicology and safety testing is conducted on new molecular entities prior to their human introduction, but companies can choose to delay long-term toxicity testing until after the therapeutic potential of the product is established.

Regulatory Review: Investigational New Drug (IND) Application

An application filed with the U.S. FDA prior to human testing.

The IND application is a compilation of all known information about the compound. It also includes a description of the clinical research plan for the product and the specific protocol for phase I study. Unless the FDA says no, the IND is automatically approved after 30 days and clinical tests can begin.

Phase I Clinical Evaluation

The first testing of a new compound in human subjects, for the purpose of establishing the tolerance of healthy human subjects at different doses, defining its pharmacologic effects at anticipated therapeutic levels, and studying its absorption, distribution, metabolism, and excretion patterns in humans.

Phase II Clinical Evaluation

Controlled clinical trials of a compound's potential usefulness and short term risks. A relatively small number of patients, usually no more than several hundred subjects, enrolled in phase II studies.

Phase III Clinical Evaluation

Controlled and uncontrolled clinical trials of a drug's safety and effectiveness in hospital and outpatient settings. Phase III studies gather precise information on the drug's effectiveness for specific indications, determine whether the drug produces a broader range of adverse effects than those exhibited in the small study populations of phase I and II studies, and identify the best way of administering and using the drug for the purpose intended. If the drug is approved, this information forms the basis for deciding the content of the product label. Phase III studies can involve several hundred to several thousand subjects.

Process Development for Manufacturing and Quality Control

Engineering and manufacturing design activities to establish a company's capacity to produce a product in large volume and development of procedures to ensure chemical stability, batch-to-batch uniformity, and overall product quality.

Bioavailability Studies

The use of healthy volunteers to document the rate of absorption and excretion from the body of a compound's active ingredients.

Companies conduct bioavailability studies both at the beginning of human testing and just prior to marketing to show that the formulation used to demonstrate safety and efficacy in clinical trials is equivalent to the product that will be distributed for sale. Companies also conduct bioavailability studies on marketed products whenever they change the method used to administer the drug (e.g., from injection or oral dose form), the composition of the drug, the concentration of the active ingredient, or the manufacturing process used to produce the drug.

Regulatory Review: New Drug Application (NDA)

An application to the FDA for approval to market a new drug. All information about the drug gathered during the drug discovery and development process is assembled in the NDA. During the review period, the FDA may ask the company for additional information about the product or seek clarification of the data contained in the application.

Postapproval Research

Experimental studies and surveillance activities undertaken after a drug is approved for marketing. Clinical trials conducted after a drug is marketed (referred to as phase IV studies in the United States) are an important source of information on as yet undetected adverse outcomes, especially in populations that may not have been involved the premarketing trials (*e.g.*, children, the elderly, pregnant women) and the drug's long-term morbidity and mortality profile. Regulatory authorities can require companies to conduct Phase IV studies as a condition of market approval. Companies often conduct post-marketing studies in the absence of a regulatory mandate.

Chapter 11

Therapeutic Innovation and Intellectual Property Rights

Drugs can be categorized according to their degree of therapeutic innovation and their status of intellectual property protection.

New Chemical Entities (NCEs) are newly developed drugs, characterized by their therapeutic innovation. An innovation may be substantial when it completely changes a therapeutic field. This is, for instance, the case with vaccines against hepatitis B because so far there is no efficient drug to cure this disease. Companies specializing in NCEs invest heavily in product research. In the USA, pharmaceutical companies' research budgets may reach over 20 per cent of their revenues. The US *Pharmaceutical Manufacturers and Research Association* (PhMRA) states a figure of US$ 500 million per NCE. In spite of the use of more rational methods the costs of *research and development* (R&D) per NCE have soared in 30 years. But the causes of this growth and the real average cost of R&D per NCE are not precisely known. In fact *DiMasi*, who published the most thorough company financed study on this point found a considerably lower figure of US$ 231 million. Yet the DiMasi study overestimates the companies' expenditures for R&D per NCE, for instance by including outlays made by public funds such as the US *National Institute of Health* (NIH).

Such debates on the cost of R&D are not merely academic, in so far as companies use them to legitimate the prices of NCEs which now are commonly 50 per cent higher than production costs. It is therefore an indispensable prerequisite for pharmaceutical industries to protect their products by intellectual property rights such as patents. In developed countries, patent protection generally lasts for a period of 20 years from the date of filing the patent. In reality, this protection period is often shorter, because regulatory approval of a drug can delay its marketing for several years after the patent is granted.

Me-too drugs are only a variation on existing drugs that are already under patent protection. The therapeutic innovation of these substances is low or zero. They have comparable medical benefits, but they circumvent patents on NCEs and allow the producers to get a share of the market. This is the case, for example, for many new products developed in industrialized countries for the treatment of hypertension.

Generics are copies of well-known drugs for which patent protection has expired. Companies specializing in generics invest little on research, or only on research in manufacturing procedures. The benefit of generics for consumers essentially lies in the price, which are usually 30 per cent below those for patent protected NCEs. All over the world, the share of the market of generics is growing. For instance, in the USA over 50 per cent of the prescriptions concern generics.

Prices and Patents

With the advent of new biotechnologies, methods for developing NCEs have changed rapidly in the last thirty years. Then, from the 1980s onwards, biotechnology also allowed new approaches in the production of drugs; genetically modified micro-organisms were employed to produce desired proteins with complex molecular structures, such as human insulin, which could not be synthesized through classical chemical methods. These changes in creating new drugs coincided with new methods in evaluating them. Mainly through the development of pharmacology the efficiency and security of new drugs can be determined with increased precision. Drug evaluation is often very time-consuming and costly. For *recombinant tissue plasminogen activator* (rTPA), a drug which is used to dissolve blood clots after acute heart infarction, two studies, each involving over 40 000 patients, were needed to prove its efficiency compared with that of an alternative drug, *streptokinase*. The heavy costs of these clinical tests bring up the question of who owns their results, once the patent is expired. In fact, the protection period for these data adds to the patent period. US law grants a protection of data for five years after the expiry of the patent before competitors can use it. In Europe this period varies in different countries, and the European Commission aims at a ten year protection rule. Pharmaceutical manufacturers have always relied on various biological methods, for instance for serum and vaccine production. However, the importance of biotechnological methods for this industry is steadily increasing. An important factor is the knowledge of the genome of both micro-organisms and humans which opens new vistas into the conception of drugs and vaccines. Should this knowledge of the genome be patented, the patent holders would have exclusive rights to its exploitation. As the UK newspaper *The Guardian* reported in May 1998, the US company *Human Genome Science* (HGS) has applied to patent one of the bacteria that causes meningitis. The application is one of three filed at the European Patent Office by HGS who are seeking to be the first to own the whole genetic sequence of bacteria. If the application is granted, as seems likely, it will open the door for commercial companies to patent any life form from which profits are expected. It could lead to royalties being paid on every treatment if a new vaccine against the illness is found. The prospect has appalled scientists in the field, who believe discoveries should be shared for the common good and that the scramble for patents for commercial gain will damage research (32).

Multinational Companies and Pharmaceutical Production in Developing Countries

In 1996 the first ten *multinational companies* (MNCs) accounted for approximately 36 per cent of the world pharmaceutical sales of US$ 251 billion. The position of MNCs in pharmaceutical production greatly differs among various developing countries.

In countries such as Brazil, Chile, Morocco, Pakistan, the Philippines, South Africa, and in Sub-Saharan Africa, national policies have invited MNCs to manufacture locally part of the drugs as a form of import-substitution policy. The biggest share of the national markets is held by MNCs who produce locally or through licensed local companies. This production is based on imported bulk chemicals. As a consequence, prices for drugs in these countries are often higher than in industrialized countries. The generated profits contribute to the research investment of MNCs, which do not meet the developing countries' most urgent needs. Pricing strategies by MNCs in these countries seem focused on the wealthier layers of the population, without any systematic price discrimination in favour of the poorer population. Some drug donations or dumpings widely advertised seem to be more cosmetic operations than basic elements in their price strategy. For instance, in March 1998 *Glaxo Wellcome* (UK) announced that it would sell its anti-HIV drug AZT for 70 per cent below the normal price to pregnant women in developing countries.

In other countries, such as Argentina, China, Egypt and India, national policy has enabled a locally financed pharmaceutical industry which is almost exclusively engaged in manufacturing generic drugs. In these countries MNCs have a weaker position. For instance in India, MNCs hold only a 20 per cent market share. Some of the national companies have important capacities in R&D aiming at manufacturing processes for already known drugs. These countries have been able to develop a bulk drug industry for antibiotics and some chemical products competitive in quality and price and export them into industrialized or other developing countries.

Table 11.1: The World's Top Ten Pharmaceutical Companies

Company	*1996 Pharmaceutical Sales (million US$)*	*Pharmaceutical Sales as per cent of Total Revenues*
Glaxo Wellcome (UK)	13,026	100
Merck & Co. (USA)	11,617	59
Novartis (Switzerland)	9,858	34
Bristol-Myers Squibb (USA)	8,702	58
Hoechst Marion Roussel (Germany)	8,652	26
Roche (Switzerland)	8,462	65
Pfizer (USA)	8,188	72
American Home Products (USA)	7,924	56
SmithKline Beecham (UK)	7,431	60
Johnson & Johnson (USA)	7,188	33

Source: Scrip's 1997 Pharmaceutical Company League Tables. RAFI Communique November/December 1997.

India is an exception because R&D efforts have also led to the development of NCEs such as vaccines against leprosy and hepatitis B, and anti-cancer drugs. In general, drug prices are very low in these countries since prices rather than innovation are the priority within the national drug policies. India holds a record, with prices for many drugs 10 to 100 times lower than in developed countries (33).

Health or Trade First?

The Uruguay Round negotiations, which concluded in 1994 with the establishment of the *World Trade Organization* (WTO), again launched a debate on the best means to foster essential drugs procurement. Within this framework, the Agreement on *Trade-Related Aspects of Intellectual Property Rights* (TRIPS) settles a minimum standard for national regulations on patents. It compels developing countries to re-write their patent regulations before the year 2000 and the least developed countries to do so before the year 2005. The Agreement sets out that patents must grant protection for at least 20 years after the date of patent application, both for *products* and *processes*. The Agreement thus settles the long-standing conflict over pharmaceutical product patents. PhMRA claimed that the US pharmaceutical industry loses US$ 500 million annually only through a lack of patent protection on drugs in India. Although many developing countries began to enforce patent protection for pharmaceutical products in the late 1980s, the majority only recognized process patents in this field. Countries like India, Argentina and those from the Middle East emphasize that this trade agreement will carry severe consequences on their national pharmaceutical industries specialized in manufacturing generics and improving production processes. It is feared that this agreement will cause an important rise of drug prices which makes them less affordable to their populations.

Other positions were based on case studies in India, arguing that the general level of drug prices will not be heavily affected, because less than 10 per cent of drugs would be under the monopoly of licensed drug manufacturers. Following this argument, all depends on the way these agreements are applied, on the accompanying measures to be taken, as well as on the policies implemented by MNC and local companies.

A careful reading of the TRIPS agreement shows that it leaves significant space to manoeuvre on different strategic points. National patent laws can serve the purpose of the WTO to spread technologies. At the same time they should protect consumers and not only inventors. For example, member states have the opportunity to exclude diagnostic and therapeutic methods for humans and animals from patenting. States can urge patent holders to license their patents in order to favour competition. For the same purpose the possibility of parallel importation is left open: a country can also import a trademark or patented product from another country where it is legally protected (35).

Governments may also have broader development concerns. Only a few developing countries are able to develop a R&D activity on drugs enabling them to create NCEs. Patent holders will therefore be in most cases foreign enterprises, and the development of national industries will depend on the willingness of these companies to license their new patented products.

As reflected by examples from India and China, the few developing countries' pharmaceutical industries which are competitve will not necessarily develop drugs targeted towards developing countries. Instead, they will probably aim at the more profitable world market, as MNCs do (36-38).

This shows the importance of a publicly funded research dedicated to meet the most urgent needs in public health. The issue on patents cannot in itself give orientation to health care research policies. Patents are unavoidable as they induce companies to innovate, but their regulations must be balanced by public health imperatives.

Chapter 12

Guide to New Entrepreneurs

As a start, we will look at what the biotechnology start-up companies do now to see why these areas have been successful and others have not.

Biotechnology investment since the mid 1970s has been in health-care, and specifically in the discovery of new drugs. An effective new drug can be sold at good profits for as long as the patent on it prevents someone else from selling it at a lower price. Once a drug comes 'off patent' it can be manufactured as a 'generic', and profit margins on it plummet. Patents do not last forever and, if a drug takes 15 years to develop, a patent will only protect its manufacturer from competition for a further 5 years. This means that the original inventor of the drug must have invented a new one every five years (ideally more often), if they are to sell high value, high profit drugs. Thus discovery or invention of new drugs is critical to the commercial strategy of many big pharmaceutical companies. In fact, the drug 'super-companies' formed by the mergers that created such companies as Glaxo-Wellcome and Novartis must launch at least three new drugs each year to keep their competitive position.

In this chapter we will summarise the application of the technologies of biotechnology to drug discovery. A wide range of discovery techniques can identify a molecular target, although genomics-based discovery is currently considered one of the most powerful. This 'target' is a molecular entity whose activity is considered important in a disease. The rest of the discovery process then searches for a small molecule compound that will interfere with the effects of that target. The result is a candidate drug, which is developed into the active ingredient of a medicine.

This process has a high failure rate–only about 4 percent of programmes succeed in producing a drug that is approved by the regulators, and probably less than 25 percent of these are profitable. And it is very expensive: a drug typically takes around $250 million to bring it to market, and most of them fail along the way (these are similar costs and success rates to a Hollywood blockbuster film, a new make of car, or re-launching Pepsi in blue cans). Typical failure rates, times and costs are which are noted is very less, but the reality is even worse than this, because you have to run at least 12 target discovery programmes at Rs.3.5 million each to have an even chance of getting one drug at the end. This means that the pharmaceutical industry spends nearly 20% of its aggregate Rs.20.9 billion 1998 R&D expenditure on things that do not work. They are therefore willing to pay very large sums to biotechnology companies that can provide science or technology that:

- Enhances the understanding of the disease (and hence lowers the inherent risk in this approach)
- Increases the efficiency of the discovery process (and hence means you can do more discovery for less cost); has already been proven in clinical trials to be superior to existing therapy.

This is a continuous of activity from basic biomedical research to commercial drug development, and the drug discovery biotechnology industry. Thus some companies essentially applied extensions of academic groups, others are indistinguishable from small drug companies. In between are companies providing specific technological skills or services, such as companies providing genomics, combinatorial chemistry, or molecular design technology, or companies specialising in screening. In addition, some companies are seeking to radically alter the order in which these steps are done, for example performing aspects of the conventional development as part of discovery.

Medical diagnostics have a quite different dynamic. While it is hard for an academic researcher to discover a new drug, it is relatively easy to discover a new diagnostic 'marker' for the difference between sick and healthy people. The limitation on their commercialisation is making them reliable and simple enough to be used on a large scale, and ideally to be performed by automated machinery, thus removing the need for skilled assay technicians. As a result, the diagnostics industry is dominated by a small number of companies with powerful marketing and distribution abilities, usually allied to their 'platform' instrumentation—large automated instruments that can perform a wide range of tests. Small companies can only gain a foothold in this market by finding specialist niches, such as specialist 'over-the-counter' tests (for pregnancy, cholesterol etc.), or unusual medical specialties that do not fit into the mainstream of diagnostics.

Genomics-driven drug discovery may change this, with drugs being increasingly targeted according to diagnostic tests that have been developed for those drugs (an idea called the RxDx tandem). This will create needs for many new technologies and systems for testing.

Biotechnology Companies: Their Care and Nurturing

The 'biotechnology company' is a company that is set up specifically to turn the science of biotechnology into a commercial product and sell the result. It is the *science* base of the company that is defining. Now, we will discuss what it takes to take a biotechnology company from that initial scientific idea to a flourishing commercial enterprise.

General Rules

Successful biotechnology companies must combine scientific creativity with market need.

Scientific Creativity

The science in a new biotechnology company generally falls into 'discovery'—you have discovered something wonderful—or 'platform technology'—you can do something wonderful. In either case, first-rate science is needed to found a first-rate company. Because living systems cannot be exactly modelled or predicted, genuinely new products must be created, at least in part, by experimental research. This must in turn be based on knowledge, creativity, and rigorous and systematic investigation, the hallmarks of good science in any context. We shall return to this theme several times, because it is crucial.

Good science is not necessarily 'leading edge' science. Research has 'fashions' and, to an extent, the biotechnology industry follows the fashion because these areas of research or technologies are where senior researchers have chosen to work. But they are not the only, or even the most productive, areas where creativity can be exercised. It can be 'old science', carried out rigorously (37).

Nor, unfortunately, does it necessarily mean science that is captivating for the bench scientist to perform. However, it must conform to what most people would recognise as scientific 'good practice'. This is taking care that your experiments test your hypothesis rigorously, and using all the data and knowledge available to put the results in context. Several high-profile failures of biotechnology companies, notably some of the early 'products' for the treatment of sepsis using monoclonal antibodies, are now recognised as being due to companies pushing poor science in order to achieve funding goals.

Market Need

Science on its own is not enough. We must sell it to someone—a 'market'. But what is 'market need'? A general statement that, for example, 'People want a cure for AIDS' is not useful. Which people? Who will pay for it? How? How much? Will your product cure all cases of AIDS or only some? Just as scientific creativity cannot occur in a vacuum, so market research must research something specific. Biotechnology research and development is expensive, so it is important that a market for the intended product is big enough to give a return on all the investment needed.

The Basic Components

The market is the environment in which the company works—it is not a component of the company. Science is a central, critical component, but it is not the only one. For the biotechnologist, it is important to remember that the scientist does not have to provide all of the other features we will discuss below, but someone does. If the team initiating a biotechnology programme cannot provide an aspect of the successful commercialisation of a piece of science, then they should team up with someone else who can. This is the role that seed venture companies can provide, as can 'business angels'—individuals who can bring their own wealth and business experience to a company as joint investors and directors.

People

A new company's need for excellent, motivated people who have commitment as well as skill and knowledge is paramount. Who is going to be the entrepreneur who makes this company happen? It may be the founding scientists, but they are not going to do it in any spare time left from an academic job. It is not going to be the scientific advisory board, who are there to advise and support the scientists. It is not going to be the Board of Directors. It needs someone to jump with both feet into the science and business and make sure that things happen.

In Europe the fear of failure has severely limited academics' inclination to do this. To a limited extent, the USA supports entrepreneurship even at the cost of failure—it is seen as meritorious to have 'had a go' and failed, because it proves motivation and drive, and the scientist who has tried and failed is unlikely to fail again in the same way, thus increasing the chances of success. In Europe, cultural conservatism means that failure is considered more significant than effort. People are therefore not willing to try for a major success if there is a significant risk of failure. This cultural barrier is disappearing slowly; the high media profile of successful scientific entrepreneurs is encouraging this cultural change and an increasing number of scientists are 'having a go'. But, in our experience, the large majority of researchers who want to see their science commercialised also are unwilling to jump whole-heartedly into that commercialisation themselves.

Although the central, driving entrepreneur is often a founding scientist with a 'good idea', it need not be. Packard Inc. were turned into a leader in the field of scientific analytical instrumentation by two business school graduates who, at the start, knew almost no science at all. Against the background of failures and successes in Europe and the USA in the last 10 years, experience shows that both business and scientific skills are essential for the success of a company, and that it is a rare scientist indeed who can combine both roles. No biotechnology company has been a commercial success when one person tried to combine both roles for more than the first 2-3 years.

Attitudes and Culture

This 'jump-in-feet-first' approach from academia requires a major culture change. Academic science focuses on the subject, commercial science on the object. Academics typically address a topic or discipline, and follow it wherever it goes. It is the process of research that is important. Commercial science addresses a specific problem, and uses any tools or disciplines that are appropriate. It is the product that is king.

These apparently small differences in emphasis have major cultural effects. For example, there is little reward for an academic to be part of a multi-disciplinary team but it is essential for most commercial programmes. It is impossible for an academic scientist to be 'redundant', as by definition what they do is what they are meant to be doing. (They may be incompetent or unfundable, but that is different.) Industrial scientists can most definitely be redundant in the sense that their science, no matter how excellent, is no longer needed to achieve the company's aims. This is made more acute by the need for a company to focus on a small number of products or projects, while it is worth an academic group having at least as many projects as it has PhD students.

This is not the same as the choice between 'blue sky' and 'applied' research. Many companies carry out highly speculative research, and much academic work in biomedicine is, in essence, applied.

Some academics believe that these differences make science, in a commercial context, less attractive to the scientist. This old-fashioned view is now not very widely held because commercial science, and especially commercial science in a small company, can be an extraordinary place to do science for several reasons:

- the environment is intellectually stimulating, with hard problems to solve and many different disciplines being brought to bear to solve them;
- problems change fast;
- money is not usually a limit in developing excellent science, and state-of-the-art equipment and materials are in plentiful supply;
- there is a real opportunity for career development into any or all of the areas of science, technology or business the

- there is the chance of making substantial financial gains from your inventiveness (although not usually a large salary in the short term in a small company).

Strategy

Having found the people, and the great science, you must decide what you are going to do. This is your strategy, what you mean to do in the longer term, beyond the exigencies of day-to-day research. The strategy of a company is, of course, specific to that company, but we can frame the things that the strategy should address as questions. Some key strategic questions for a small company start-up are:

- What is your company's specific aim? 'Cure cancer' is not a reasonable strategic goal for a health-care company.
- What is your first product going to be? This is absolutely essential. Out of the cornucopia that your science could create, you must choose one thing to start with and focus most of your energies on that one. This 'focus' is critical for new science-driven companies. This means hard choices and it means dumping some 'pet projects'.
- How do you deal with success? Success in a research programme usually means having to start a development programme. Do you have the skills or funds to do this? If not, how are you going to get them?
- What will you do next? After your initial research programme has finished (with success or failure), do you have to fire all the scientists or do you have another programme for them to move on to? Remember that a company's science is focused on a particular problem, not on a discipline or process. Whatever those scientists have to do, it must fit in with the overall aims of the company and the company's competitive advantage. Define what the key scientific advantage of the company is and hence what the scientists are going to be doing.

Do not confuse 'strategy' with 'mission statement'. The latter is a single phrase that encapsulates what you think you are about but it says nothing about why, how, or what you are going to do to get there. Some people think 'mission statements' are purely public relationship exercises for the company brochure.

Product vs. Service vs. Technology

A key aspect of your strategy is how your company is going to make money. In the 1980s it was every biotechnology company's stated dream to become a FIPCO—a 'Fully Integrated Pharmaceutical Company', like Pfizer or Roche, doing everything from basic discovery to trucking boxes of pills to doctors. This is very unrealistic (31).

There are several more realistic goals:

Product Company

You discover or invent products, take them as far through development as your funding allows, and then sell or license them to someone with experience in manufacture, distribution, etc. Examples include all the larger 'first wave' biotech companies such as Amgen, Celltech and Chiroscience. In rare cases, these companies may seek to manufacture their own product. In even rarer ones they may go round doctor's surgeries selling it. But there are probably 400,000 general practitioners in Europe alone. Are you going to personally sell your pills to them all? If not, someone must work with you on that end of the business.

Tools Company

You develop tools or technologies that help other people develop products. Examples of such 'toolsets' include genomics and combinatorial chemistry. These are often also called 'technology platform' companies.

'Solution Providers'

You integrate several tools into one company. This is often achieved by the merger of two or more companies as any one start-up company may be excellent at one technique or approach but is unlikely to master all the 'tools' that a collaborator needs. Mergers and acquisitions are becoming more common in biotechnology and are an effective way of welding a lot of small brilliant companies into one (hopefully brilliant) whole. If this is your goal, you should say so from the start.

Your strategy as to which of these companies you wish to emulate will probably change. But you should at least have some idea today as the approaches the different companies take to product discovery and development are radically different, and it is that first product that will make or break your new company.

Success

Success is hard to define. Intellectual leadership is not the same as company success. A strategy must be careful to define 'success' in a useful, meaningful way. What is your ultimate goal? (Remember 'cure cancer' or 'enhance shareholder value' are too vague to be useful.) What are significant steps along the way, and how will you show that you have passed them to the outside world? Defining criteria for success is very important, as it defines your commercial goals, and hence shapes your strategy in getting there.

By different criteria, the biotechnology industry as a whole either has been very successful or a dismal failure. Less than 1 percent of the first tier of (almost all US) biotechnology companies have become profitable on the basis of sales of products. However over 90 percent are still in existence as active, science-based companies. Over 60 percent would have given their initial investors an IRR of over 10 percent ('IRR' is 'Internal Rate of Return', a measure of the financial success of the investment). For your start-up, these might be rather long-term goals. You might define success in terms of milestones along the way, such as flotation on a public stock market, signing a major collaboration with a pharmaceutical company, or entering your first product into Phase II clinical trials.

Competitive Advantage

This is a trendy phrase from the management manuals of the 1980s that means that you can do something better than your competitors. What is it that you can do and no-one else (or, more realistically, very few other people) can do? What is it that, rather than merely being good at, you *excel* at? 'Excellence' is the watchword here, and it may come from one of five reasons.

You Hold the Patent on Doing It

This is a powerful argument. Scientists should always patent an idea, process or invention that they think might be of some use to someone. The patent prohibits anyone else from 'practising' your patented invention without your agreement. It does not physically prevent anyone from copying your invention, but it makes it illegal to do so, and you can sue them if you have the time and money, and it is worth the effort. An example is the patent on polymerase chain reaction owned by Hoffman-La Roche, to whom anyone in the world using PCR for commercial purposes must pay a license fee or Roche will sue them.

You Have the Tools Necessary to Do It

This is as good as holding the patent in the short term, as it means that, while someone else could copy your process or invention in theory, in practice they cannot. Examples would be owning key cell lines, gene clones or production equipment. This, however, is only a competitive advantage until your competitors can either duplicate your tools, or find a way round using them, for example, by building their own production plant. A good tool to own is therefore one that inherently cannot be duplicated, like a unique genetic population.

You Have the Skills Necessary to Do It

Early practitioners in the science of *in vitro* fertilisation were in that position, as are those able to produce clones of mammals from adult cells today. This is a powerful competitive weapon until someone else learns how to do it. The skills base of this sort is sometimes called the company's 'intellectual capital'.

You Have a Lot of Resources or Money to Do It

This is a weaker form of competitive advantage in biotechnology, because the industry is a knowledge-based one, not a resources based one. Many companies have lots of resources, especially major pharmaceutical or agricultural companies, and if your sole competitive advantage is that you have bought 20 DNA synthesisers and lots of computers and technicians to run them then you will shortly be out-competed by another company which can afford 30 DNA synthesisers.

You are the First to Do It

This is the least attractive of all but it is often where biotechnology companies start. They see an opportunity and set up a company to exploit it. Their advantage is that they can move faster than anyone else. This only lasts while you keep moving.

Other forms of competitive advantage that apply to companies, such as Pepsico or Ford, such as having efficient factories or a recognised 'brand name', rarely apply to biotechnology companies.

The only way to show you have a competitive advantage is to demonstrate that what you want to do can actually work. In therapeutics discovery, this means proving that your material has some effect in people (remember that most drug discovery programmes fail). As it takes tens of millions of pounds or dollars to develop a product to the point of proving therapeutic efficacy, companies often have to accept a less rigorous proof, such as a sound scientific reason for supposing that it will work, evidence from animal tests that it works in animals, evidence that it is not actually harmful in humans (Phase I data).

Competitive Intelligence

Part of proving that you have a competitive advantage is knowing how good you are compared to how good you have to be. This is competitive intelligence. Is there a medical need that you are going to satisfy and is someone else already filling that need? Is that need still going to be there in 10 years' time? This is a combination of finding out what the competition is doing, and what the market is. A surprising number of business proposals we have seen contain no evidence that their authors realise that the outside world exists, even less that it might contain competitors.

The Business Plan

Many of the rules for success go beyond 'strategy' and into tactics. Tactical planning should be carried out by a team of people bringing scientific, product development, business and financial skills, because all of these things are essential. The end product of this planning is a detailed plan of what your business is going to do—a business plan. But the business plan is a *product of planning*, not an end in itself. No matter how colourful or typographically creative it is, it is worthless if the planning behind it is not rigorous.

During the construction of a business plan, scientists must be aware that not only will bankers, accountants and the like be telling them what experiments they can and cannot do in the company, but that these people actually have a valid and useful viewpoint, and can sharpen and focus a company's plan substantially. (The decision on what is and is not good science, though, must rest with the scientists unless the bankers have post-doctoral laboratory experience, which is rare.) Typically, the stages that this process goes through are summarised below: we have considered several of them already.

- Identifying the science that will go into the company, according to the criteria we summarised above.
- Defining what you are going to do with that science. This is the first part of the 'business plan', a document that should literally describe what the business plans to do. It should include consideration of

1. What can the science *really* do?
2. Who is going to do it, and where?
3. Who is going to manage them (*i.e.* make sure that everything happens)? are there bits the company cannot do, or it is not sensible to do, and if so who is going to do them, and how will you pay them?
4. Who will own the new intellectual property?
5. Who will manage the development programmes?
6. What are the key milestones?
7. Identifying the company's competitive advantage.
8. How will the company be funded, and specifically?
9. How much money do you need to get started?
10. Where will you be when that runs out, and who will give you some more then?
11. Who do you sell your product to, and by implication, what is your product? Is your strategy to generate intellectual property that you sell to another company, to develop drugs to Phase II clinical trials and then sell them to a drug company, to provide a service, or to get a product all the way to selling it to a high-street store. These paths take very different skills, and very different amounts of money.

And most importantly:

12. What happens if (when) it doesn't work?

The last point can be hard for some scientists to accept but it is a fact that most science fails and you have to ask what happens to your company then. If it is a 'one product company' then when the product fails, the company fails, and everyone is out of a job. So it is wise to look round for other technologies you can bring in to the company. It is possible that, after a year, half of the brilliant science that led to forming the company has been abandoned! This should be viewed as evidence of growth and evolution, not failure, providing it has been replaced by something better.

The whole process boils down to identifying the shortest route between where you are and where you want to go (but not taking scientifically unjustified shortcuts), with suitable cut-outs for when it does not work. This is why the strategy is important—you cannot define the shortest path to where you want to be until you know where that is. It also shows that in a company you cannot separate science from business issues.

The result of this process is a detailed plan of what the business will be doing, why it will survive and, preferably, flourish if given a certain amount of money. This forms the basis of an investment proposal—you take the plan to a funder, and say 'I propose you invest in this company because it will do this with the money'.

The business plan will almost certainly be wrong. Unforeseen events, from scientific breakthroughs or failures to stock market crashes, will derail your carefully laid plans. This should be expected, even embraced. But if you cannot think through where you might go if all goes well, the chances are that you will go nowhere.

Investment in Biotechnology

Having defined what your company is to do, you need money to allow you to start. Very few biotechnology ideas can be realised in a way that requires no investment. Sometimes the investment is 'only' a few tens of thousands of pounds (or dollars or ecus) to make the first material you can sell. More usually it will take tens or hundreds of millions. Very few individuals can afford such sums, so you must convince other people to put money into your idea. These other people are the investors. There are several different types of investor depending on the stage your company is at and they will fund you in stages. Understanding this path and the motivations of the people that you will meet along its way is important if you are to get your biotechnology company funded.

An investor should not only be a source of funding. From an early stage, the investor should also help you found and run the business. They should provide help with issues such as employment contracts, location, finding funding for expensive equipment, securing the intellectual property and having discussions (or arguments) with all the other parties involved such as university technology transfer officers, patent lawyers, and the many researchers at the founding institution who have not had the courage to do this themselves but now want a piece of the action. All this can be pushed on to the business co-founder.

Seed Investment

An increasingly common route to developing an idea into a company (which includes all the processes is to seek seed funding.

Seed funding provides enough money to set the company up, acquire key patents, negotiate the graceful exit of the founding scientists from their current job and create a corporate entity. It also pays for planning and writing the business plan, a time consuming and skill-intensive business, often in terms of the investor's time and involves hiring lawyers, patent agents and accountants. Such seed funding is provided by private investors or specialist, professional seed funding companies, which are still rare in Europe, although more common in the USA. There is a general dearth of seed funding to take potential companies from 'I have this great idea' to 'This is a company you can believe in'. In part this is because the risks at this stage are huge and the rewards very uncertain. Merlin Ventures is the largest dedicated seed funding enterprise in Europe (as of mid 1998), and in two years we were able to seed only eight of the hundreds of companies that probably lie nascent in the British research establishment alone.

Private Funding for Biotechnology

Once you have a company it will probably need substantial amounts of money to pursue its product development goals. Start-up companies are usually funded privately, through investment by private transactions between the company and individuals or groups of individuals. Typically, such investments are through the issue of new shares, so new investors become shareholders and all the previous shareholders are *'diluted'* (*i.e.* have their share in the company reduced). Once the company exists, it can receive more substantial funding to carry out its plans as articulated in its business plan. This 'first round finance' (seed funding does not count as real money) comes from one of two sources:

Private investors: These are people with sufficient wealth to be able to put substantial amounts (usually at least $250,000) into the company, take some active part in helping the company in financial or commercial terms and, most importantly, take the risk that they will lose their investment.

Venture capitalists (VC): These are people or companies who specialise in investment in risky propositions, usually early stage companies. They set up a fund into which people put their money and then the venture capital 'fund managers' invest that in high-risk ventures. This is exactly analogous to the investment trusts and funds that are common savings routes for the general public but with far higher risks and, the investors hope, far higher returns.

Both types of investor will want to check your business over for criteria which include the people involved, their 'due diligence' study on the science, the return on investment, exit route, and whether anyone else is willing to fund the idea.

People

Most VC groups will invest in people as much as in science. This is because the science on which a company is founded will almost certainly go wrong, and when it does it is the people who will either put it right or give up. The former is preferable. How someone goes about this is as much a matter of their general experience and personality as the specifics of the programme they want to get funded. 'Good' things in the scientific founders of a company are a *demonstrated* willingness to change fields, learn new expertise, collaborate with people from different disciplines, think of lateral things to do when challenged. A desire to make a lot of money is also good and a desire to be famous is usually bad, because it often ends up as being famous at the expense of the company rather than to its benefit.

Often a VC will also look for 'management', specifically a Chief Executive Officer (CEO). This person will have experience in running a science-based, commercial operation of some sort, will be accepted by the scientists as their company leader and is a credible person to put in front of bankers, accountants and other city professionals. A few VCs can perform the role of 'the suit' themselves (Merlin Ventures can, and does, for example), but most will not be willing to run the day-to-day operations of the dozen companies in their portfolio, and so will insist on at least a skeleton management being in the company from the start. This role can be played by the business angel or other seed investor.

Due Diligence

After assuring themselves that the people are at least potentially suitable, the VC will carry out an external test of the science, by calling up experts, having any patents checked out by lawyers, asking around at meetings and conferences, and checking the perceived strength of the company's science, technology and people. This is known as 'due diligence' (after a legal phrase meaning in essence 'I have done whatever I can'). Due diligence can vary from a few chats in a bar to a full-scale consultancy project costing hundreds of thousands of pounds.

The due diligence process gives the VC an estimate for how reliable the current science is and what the market might be. Usually this will differ materially from the scientists' view. It is critical for the calculation of the 'value' of the company today, and hence a calculation of the Return on Investment (ROI, also sometimes called the Internal Rate of Return—IRR). This is the amount of money they will get out compared to the amount they put in, and is usually expressed as a percentage annual growth rate (like a bank might offer eight percent to its savers). VCs usually look for ROIs of 50 percent per annum or more: this is not greed (or not only greed), but reflects the fact that this is the ROI they will get if everything works—usually, of course, it does not and they get an ROI of less than zero percent.

It is also worthwhile for an entrepreneur to do 'due diligence' on the VC to see what they have done for people in the past, in terms of help with management, guidance in business and scientific strategy, building the company up so it can cope with its own success and contacts in the world of finance. Most say that they can do this, although it is the sad truth that few do.

Exit Route

No-one putting money into a start-up biotechnology company expects to be paid back from the company's profits, at least for a minimum of 5 years, so there must be some other 'exit route' by which they get their money back. This can be

- Privately selling your share in the company to someone else;
- Getting bought by another company (merger or acquisition being different versions of a similar process);
- Floating on the stock exchange (when the company is big and stable enough) and so in effect selling your shares to the general public.

All are possible for any company, if they are successful, so the question here is when will it happen. The 'when' is critical for calculation of ROI—a 100 percent gain in value in one year is 100 percent per annum ROI: a 200 percent gain in 4 years is a 50 percent ROI, even though the absolute amount of the latter is higher.

Funding Stages

VCs usually invest when a company has already gained some seed funds, has developed its business plan, hired a couple of people, but has not got seriously under way. This is known as 'first round' or 'first stage' finance, and is typically between £0.5 million and £3 million. This is the riskiest end of venture capital. This money will typically take a company engaged in drug discovery and development through 1.5 to 3 years' work, and take the science from some basic research to a proof of principle. Then the company will need to raise more money, arranged in a second round finance with companies that specialise in that stage of investment. Second stage finance houses tend to lean more heavily on formal due diligence studies, look for an experienced management team in place, and look to the detailed timing of when they can float the company and so get their money back. Second round funding usually raises between £8 million and £15 million.

If all goes well, the company will then be floated on a stock exchange in another two or three years. This should raise £10-30 million. However it may need a 'top-up' funding to get it there—this is termed Mezzanine financing. Alternatively, things may go wrong with the science, requiring another round of private funding.

Corporate Partners

The other main source of funds for your new company is other companies, and usually much larger ones. These may be clients (*i.e.* ones who buy your products) but, in the early days, most biotech companies have no products. So larger companies may become partners with you in order to help you develop products. They benefit because you have something that can help them innovate. You benefit because they provide skills or infrastructure you do not have, such as the problem alluded to previously of distributing. Often corporate partners will also fund, organise and perform later stage clinical trials (which can be hugely expensive and complicated) as well.

In essence a corporate partner is a combination of collaborator and client. You get funds and resources, they get new programmes or products.

There are a huge variety of corporate partnership arrangements, from simple purchase of goods to outright purchase of the company. However the things that corporate partners will look for in your company are surprisingly similar to those a VC will look for, Bear in mind that few companies have all of these—however if your start-up has *none* of them, you will have some problems getting it funded.

Grants

Occasionally agencies that provide grants to academics to perform research will also provide grants to biotechnology companies. However much more common is other types of government grant support aimed at such 'SMEs' (Small to Medium-sized Enterprises). The biotechnology industry is knowledge-based, clean, rapidly growing, and based in the West's long investment in its scientific and technological infrastructure. Also, much of it is addressing healthcare, probably the only sector of the economy to grow every decade this century. So biotechnology is seen as 'good', both socially and economically, and is encouraged with various degrees of vigour by governments.

This has led to a profusion of types of government support for new biotechnology from which start-up companies can benefit. These include:

Technology Transfer Schemes

These are schemes to help transfer science or technology from (usually) a university setting into a commercial one. Following US models, European technology transfer offices are now becoming better equipped and better skilled to find the most appropriate route for commercialisation.

Small Company Support Schemes

Such as SMART and SPUR in the UK. These are generic schemes to help small companies get off the ground with government financial assistance.

Regional Development Support

This is government support to try to encourage industry to settle in one region rather than another. Only occasionally are these places where the best science and scientists are already based.

National and International Co-ordination Efforts

These are attempts to get the technology policy or regional support geographically integrated. There are some commercially based schemes, such as EUREKA to encourage pan-European commercial developments.

Major Infrastructure Programmes with Biotechnology Relevance

In both Europe and the USA the government supports major programmes of work which have biotechnology spin-offs, such as genome projects. These are usually 'pre-competitive'.

These can provide very substantial sums for companies especially if they are in areas of Europe targeted for economic development such as Liverpool or Sicily. However it is generally true that if the company is depending on grants to survive, then it was a bad economic idea from the start.

The Stock Market and Biotechnology

More established companies can raise money from the general public by selling shares on a stock market, where suitably regulated brokers trade shares on behalf of their clients. Public funding in this way has very different constraints from private funding. It is very closely regulated to stop companies or brokers defrauding the public.

Shareholders have statutory rights that mean that they are the ultimate arbiters of the company's future, and many company brochures will talk about 'increasing shareholder value' as recognition that these people actually own the company. In principle shareholders can fire the board of directors, or demand the company accounts for its actions, although in practice only major investment funds, which hold large blocks of shares, are in a position to exert any control over how the company is run.

In order to get a biotechnology company 'listed' (*i.e.* have their name put on the list of shares available for trade), the company has to demonstrate that it is suitably stable. In the developed countries like UK this means having a trading record for several years, or having at least two products in clinical trials, or a number of other criteria. It also means having a prospectus that has been verified by lawyers to say that every statement in it is demonstrably true, even down to the definition of chemical or medical terms. Part of this process requires an external group of experts to write a report on the company, which in essence says that they, experts in the field, agree that what the company says makes sense—this is known (unsurprisingly) as 'the experts' report'. Accounts have to be presented and audited, company directors have to sign legal forms that they are suitable people, and have to be checked out for past fraud offences and so on. This is all to protect the public from the worst excesses of entrepreneurship.

When and where you float your company is an arcane art. There are many different stock markets that can list a company, and listing in market one does not imply listing in any of the others, as they all have slightly different rules and constituencies. Although their enthusiasm for biotechnology investments waxes and wanes roughly in unison, there can be substantial differences.

Valuing Biotechnology Companies

Public and private financing is by selling shares in your company. In essence, you sell a part of the company to someone in exchange for funds. But what are your shares worth? If someone is willing to give you £4 million, does this buy five percent of your company, or 95 percent? It depends on whether your company is worth £80 million or £4.2 million. Valuing your company appropriately is therefore important.

The details of how a value is placed on a company is beyond the scope of this article. In summary:

- There is no rational way of valuing a start-up company. You have some ideas, some patents, some people, and no premises, products, established programmes or track record. The overwhelming objective factor is the chance that your crucial first product will fail, scientifically or commercially, and this probability is a matter of opinion. Values are dominated by 'feel' and your credibility.

➤ When the company has been in business 3-4 years, has 40 employees and two products in late development, we can 'guesstimate' its value by working out what the company will be worth when it reaches its final goal and the chances it will make it there. Your goal may be to be bought out for $550 million or to generate a stream of new drugs that you will sell to a big pharmaceutical company. This gives you a final figure, and a guess for how long it will take to get there. You then multiply this by the probability of achieving it (<<1), divide it by return that you could have earned investing money in a 'safe' investment over the same time (>1), and that is your value.

If you are a public company, your value is the number of outstanding shares multiplied by whatever people will pay for them. This can lead your company to suddenly losing value because the share price drops and is the reason that reporters say that falls in the stock market have 'wiped billions off the value of industry'.

Who Needs Management?

'Management' is a word that has come up several times in the previous sessions. Why are investors so keen on management?

The scale of operations of a company is larger than in a research group. A drug discovery and development company can expect to grow to 30-50 people in 18 months, to over 100 people in 3 years, all working on essentially the same product or related groups of products. This cannot happen by chance—it must be organised. It must also be focused on a very specific goal. Company funding is based on success not on activity. If a line of research is not working someone has to make the hard decisions about what to do about it including, *in extremis*, firing the scientists involved.

This needs professional management—people who know how to organise and run a scientific programme with such defined goals. Sometimes the scientists can grow into this role. Sometimes they can accept it from an outsider recruited to the company specifically to manage it. But filling that role is an absolute condition of setting up a company, and companies without effective management almost always fail. Sometimes they take a long time and a lot of money to fail, which is why investors look for good management as part of the company team: without it, there is a very high probability that their money will be wasted.

This imposition of management is sometimes resented by scientists used to academic freedom, because they feel that they are 'giving up control' of their science. This is a fallacy for three reasons:

1. They are not giving up control of anything—before the company was founded there was nothing there to control. No-one was developing the product, hiring the scientists, performing the work.
2. It is not 'their' science. A successful company must be assembled from many scientific and technical strands, for reasons outlined in the previous sessions. They are a contributor, not a sole author.
3. No one person is in control of a small company, if it is to perform with the energy, flexibility and enthusiasm that will carry it to success. It must be a team, not a dictatorship.

Where is Management?

Finding appropriate management is difficult. You need quite different sorts of people at different stages of a company. The senior management, and particularly the Chief Executive Officer (CEO), of a new start-up with 10 employees must be able and willing to do everything, to do without formal reporting structures, and to know everything that goes on in the company. The manager of a public company of 400 employees must delegate nearly all of that and instead control a reporting and responsibility system that has several layers between him and the bench scientist. A company's management becomes more obvious, more structured and includes more people as the company grows.

As a company grows, the people who ran the company very well at one stage have to give way to ones who are competent to run it in the next. One of the skills of the entrepreneur who starts a small company is to know when their skills should be replaced by someone suited to run a more mature organisation.

Finding people who can perform these tasks, and particularly the many-sided and changing task of running a new start-up company, is hard. As in science, the only evidence that you can do it is a 'track record' of having done it before. The CEO is particularly critical, as he has overall responsibility for making the company work. CEOs for new biotechnology companies come from a variety of backgrounds, where their experience in management, in directing science and in relating to the needs and concerns of the board of a company fit them for the role. Academic research does not usually fit a scientist for such a role. Neither does being a management consultant (criticising how someone is performing is not the same as performing well yourself), nor does 'experience' of business gained solely through an MBA (Masters of Business Administration) course.

Critical tests for a CEO of a new biotechnology start-up could be caricatured as:

The 'Nature' Test

This test can they read Nature and understand what they are reading? This is critical, as the fundamental of the start-up is good science.

The Lightbulb Test

This test can they (and are they willing to) change the lightbulb if it blows, i.e. do anything practical needed to keep the company running. There may be no-one else around to fix it.

The Cat-Herder Test

This test can they convince a group of disparate scientists that what the CEO wants them to do is more worthwhile in scientific terms than what the scientists thought they wanted to do? (He or she can threaten to fire them but that will not capture the creativity and dedication of which the best scientists are capable.)

The Deal Test

This test can the CEO go out and make deals that will bring the company money in return for a small amount of its technology of products? Such deals are critical for funding, but also to show that someone else has faith in you.

The Suit Test

This test can the CEO put on a metaphorical (or literal) dark suit and convince investors that he or she is really on their side, so their investment is safe in his or her hands?

These general criteria apply to all the senior people in a small company. The 'head of molecular biology' in a start-up may find themselves watching the pilot plant or presenting to an investment banker who does not know what DNA stands for; there are few well-defined job descriptions in such an environment. This is half the fun of it.

As well as people who run the company as a whole, your start-up will need more specialist management functions such as financial and personnel management. Initially these will be provided by someone outside the company, such as the venture capital company backing the company, or by the CEO in his 'spare time'. As the company develops, a more specialised type of manager with less concern for science and more concern for management as a process and skill in its own right is needed. Scientists should note that these people *are needed*: they are not hired purely to make your life at the bench harder. Without them you might wake up one day and find that the company has run out of money.

This brings us into the realm of general management theory and practice, which this seminar will not discuss further. There are many books and courses on this available, some of them relevant to the unique environment of a small, science-based company.

Directors and Others

In law, every company must have a Board of Directors. These people do exactly what their name implies—they direct the company so that its value to its shareholders is maximised. There are stringent laws about what company directors can and cannot do in general terms, and some financial scandals in major companies have involved directors abusing their position for their own gain.

The directors should add substantial value to the company, in terms of contacts, experience, advice and business acumen. Their role should emphatically not be just to rubber stamp what the CEO wants to do and for that reason it is considered bad practice for the Chairman of the Board to be the CEO. A venture capitalist looking to fund a company or a scientist looking to join it at a senior level will look at the Board to see whether they are there as window dressing or whether they will really help the company flourish.

Parallel to the Board, and often answering to it, most biotechnology companies have a Scientific Advisory Board (SAB). It should advise the CEO and directors on any technical aspect that the company needs guidance over and, specifically, provide perspective, contacts and advice on all areas of science that might be relevant to the company. For example, an agricultural genetics company might have an agrochemicals expert and a farmer among theirs.

Patents and Therapeutic Proteins

Patents are critical to a small company based on knowledge. If you make an invention and it is not patented, anyone with suitable resources is free to come along and copy it. For a small company, many of your competitors will have far greater resources than you do and so can simply take your ideas and use them themselves. For this reason, investors and professional management are very eager to protect your intellectual property (IP) with suitable legal walls, and ideally with patents.

The process of patenting in the UK is beyond this seminar. In summary, the scientist, advised by someone who knows the language and law of patenting, has to submit ('file') a description of the invention to the patent office. The office's own examiners then check that the patent fulfils the three critical criteria:

Novelty

No-one has done it before, or even talked about it in a realistic way.

Utility

It must be useful for something. This means that the gene you discovered is not patentable in its own right but must be related to a product.

Enablement

You must describe how someone else could do it (whatever it is).

If it passes, then the patent is granted. The process takes a long time, and costs a lot of money. In a novel field like biotechnology there is also a lot of debate (much of it carried out in the law courts) about just what 'an invention' is.

The critical part of the patent is the *exact* wording of the claims. The claims are a set of statements, usually at the end of the patent, which define exactly what it is you are patenting. If your claims are very 'broad' (*i.e.* general), you can succeed in getting a patent on a number of potential applications of your idea, not only one. The wording here is critical. Thus 'a nucleic acid' is broader than 'DNA' or 'a gene'; 'a molecule' is broader than 'an alcohol' which is broader than '2-methyl-butan-l-ol' and so on. Of course, if your claim is too broad then the patent office will not allow it because it will not be novel: use of 2-methylbutan-l-ol as a cure for cancer may be novel but use of 'a molecule' certainly is not.

Your role in patenting is therefore to make sure that you have described your invention in terms of a final product—in the case of a gene sequence, may be a diagnostic test for a genetic defect or a drug that blocks the action of that gene's protein product—and in terms that meet the criteria above. A good patent agent can be very helpful in this process and their help should be encouraged.

Conclusion: Jumping the Fence

An entrepreneur is someone who can see a way to make all the things we describe in this learning experience actually happen, and does it. The former needs knowledge, breadth of experience and contacts, but the latter is the most important, and really can be summed up in three words—Just Do It. Three words do not a seminar make, so we have focused on what an entrepreneur or business person should do to create a successful biotechnology business rather than the personal characteristics that make a scientist into an entrepreneur. But without the will to make it happen, none of this is relevant. This is why we have returned many times to the nature of the people involved rather than a formal process that will lead them gently and inevitably to success.

This is an extremely favourable time in history for new, fast-moving companies in high technology. Investors, regulators and governments all want to see your small company succeed. It is also a time of unprecedented technological change in the life sciences, and so the environment has never been better to build a life-science based company. For all its commercial failings and public misconception, the biotechnology industry will continue to be as dynamic and exciting a business sector as any in the next decade. It is a superb environment for a scientist to enter, for good science, the potential of substantial reward, and just plain fun.

References

1. Adams, M. D., Dubnick, M., Kerlavage, A. R., Moreno, R., Kelley, J. M., Utterback, T. R., Nagle, J. W., Fields, C. & Venter, J. C. (1992) Sequence Identification of 2,375 Brain Genes. *Nature*, 355 (6361), 632-4.
2. Alberts, B., Bray, D., Lewis, J., Raff, M., Roberts, K. & Watson, J. (1989) The Molecular Biology of the Cell (2nd. ed. ed.). New York, NY: Garland Publishing.
3. Buss, L. (1987) The Evolution of Individuality. Princeton, NJ: Princeton University Press.
4. Cherty, L. M., Case, S. M. & Wilson, A. C. (1978) Frog Perspectives on the Morphological difference between Humans and Chimpanzees. *Science*, 200, 209-211.
5. Doolittle, R. F., Hunkapiller, M. W., Hood, L. E., Devare, S. G., Robbins, K. C., Aaronson, S. A., & Antoniades, H. N. (1983) Simian Sarcoma Onc Gene, v-sis, Is Derived from the Gene (or Genes) Encoding Platelet Derived Growth Factor. *Science*, 221, 275-277.
6. Doubet, S., Bock, K., Smith, D., Albersheim, P. & Darvill, A. (1989) The Complex Carbohydrate Structure Database. *Trends in Biochemical Sciences*, 14, 475.
7. George, D., Barker, W. & Hunt, L. (1986) The Protein Identification Resource. *Nucleic Acids Research*, 14, 11-15.

8. Hamm, G. & Cameron, G. (1986) The EMBL Data Library. *Nucleic Acids Research*, 14, 5-9.

9. Hartwell, L. (1991) Twenty-five Years of Cell Cycle Genetics. *Genetics*, 129 (4), 975-980.

10. Hochachka, P. W. & Somero, G. N. (1984) Biochemical Adaptation. Princeton, NJ: Princeton University Press.

11. Karplus, M. & Petsko, G. A. (1990) Molecular Dynamics Simulations in Biology. *Nature*, 347 (October), 631-639.

12. Kessel, R. G. & Kardon, R. H. (1979) Tissues and Organs: A Text-Atlas of Scanning electron Microscopy. San Francisco, CA: W.H. Freeman and Company.

13. Langton, C., eds. (1989) Artificial Life (VI.). Redwood City, CA: Addison Wesley.

14. Lawton, J., Burks, C. & Martinez, F. (1989) Overview of the LiMB Database. *Nucleic Acids Research*, 17, 5885-5899.

15. Letovsky, S. & Berlyn, M. (1992) CPROP: A Rule-based Program for Constructing a Genetic Map. *Genomics*, 12, 435-446.

16. Li, W.-H. & Graur, D. (1991) Fundamentals of Molecular Evolution. Sunderland, MA: Sinauer Associates, Inc.

17. Margolis, L. (1981) Symbiosis and Cell Evolution. San Francisco: Freeman.

18. May, R. M. (1988) How Many Species Are There on Earth? Science, 241 (September 16), 1441- 1450.

19. Miyazawa, S. (1990) DNA Data Bank of Japan: Present Status and Future Plans. *Computers and DNA*, 7, 47-61.

20. Moore, J., Benton, D. & Burks, C. (1990) The GenBank Nucleic Acid Data Bank. Focus, 11 (4), 69-72.

21. Ptashne, M. (1987) A Genetic Switch: Gene Control and the Phage Lambda. Palo Alto, CA: Blackwell Scientific Publications.

22. Sauer, R. T. (1989) Genetic Analysis of Protein Stability and Function. *Annual Review of Genetics*, 23, 289-310.

23. Ulrich, E., Markley, J. & Kyogoku, Y. (1989) Creation of Nuclear Magnetic Resonance Data Repository and Literature Base. *Protein Sequence and Data Analysis*, 2, 23-37.

24. Woese, C. R., Kandler, O. & Wheelis, M. L. (1990) Towards a Natural System of Organisms: Proposal for the Domains Archaia, Bacteria, and Eucarya. (June), 4576-4579.

25. R.M. Akers, et al., (1994) Recombinant DNA Technology, vol. 2: Special Issue of Annals of the New York Academy of Science, vol. 721, pp. 218-233.

26. D E Baker, (2001) "Pegylated interferons", Rev. Gastroenterol. Disord., 1, pp. 87-99.

27. R M Bukowski, C Tendler, D Cutler, E Rose, M M Laughlin and P Statkevich, (2002) "Treating cancer with PEG Intron: pharmacokinetic profile and dosing guidelines for an improved interferon-alpha-2b formulation", *Cancer*, 95, pp. 389-396.

28. L Johnson and P Herbert (2003), "Long acting protein formulations–ProLease technology", Modified-release drug delivery technology, (Eds M J Rathbone, J Hadgraft and M S Roberts), Marcel Dekker, Inc., New York, pp. 671-677.

29. H Bentz, (2002) "Stability of non-aqueous formulations of macromolecules developed for long-term in vivo delivery", Protein and peptide drug delivery: Scientific advances enabling novel approaches & improved products, IBC Meeting, Boston, 26-27 Sept.

30. F W Okumu, L N Dao, P J Fielder, N Dybdal, D Brooks, S Sane and J L Cleland, (2002) "Sustained delivery of human growth hormone from a novel gel system: SABER", *Biomaterials*, 23, pp. 4,353-4,358.

31. Congress of the United States, Office of Technology Assessment. Pharmaceutical R&D: Costs, Risks and Rewards: 1993; pp. 4-5. Based on Pharmaceutical Manufacturers Association Annual Survey

32. Jérôme Dumoulin (1998) The role of pharmaceuticals and patents K. Bala, O. Lanza and S.R. Kaur, "Retail Drug prices: The Law of the Jungle". HAInews, nr. 100.

33. R. Ballance, J. Pogany and H. Forstner (1992) The World's Pharmaceutical Industries. An International Perspective on Innovation, Competition and Policy, prepared for the United Nations Industrial Development Organisation. Cheltenham, UK: Edward Elgar Publishing.

34. J.A. DiMasi, R.W.Hansen, H.G. Grabowski, et al. (1991) "The cost of Innovation in the Pharmaceutical Industry, *Journal of Health Economics* 10: 107-1421.

35. South Centre (1997) The TRIPs Agreement. A Guide for the South; The Uruguay Round Agreement on Trade-Related Intellectual Property Rights. Geneva, Switzerland: South Centre.

36. US Congress, Office of Technology Assessment (1993) Pharmaceutical R and D: Cost, risks and rewards. OTA-H-522. Washington DC, USA: Government Printing Office.

37. World Health Organization (1988) The World Drug Situation. Geneva, Switzerland: WHO.

38. J.I. Gallin, I.M. Goldstein, R. (1992) Snyderman, editors: Inflammation. Basic principles and clinical correlates, ed 2, New York, Raven Press

39. J.S. Warren (1990) Interleukins and tumor necrosis factor in inflammation. *Crit Rev Clin Lab Sci* 28, 37-59.

40. C.A. Dinarello (1992) Reduction of inflammation by decreasing production of interleukin-1 or by specific receptor antagonism. *Int J Tiss Reac* 14, 65-75 .

41. C.A. Dinarello (1994) Interleukin-1. In: The cytokine handbook. Ed: Thomson A., Academic Press, San Diego, .

42. J. Vilcek, T.H. Lee (1991) Tumor necrosis factor. *J Biol Chem* 266, 7313-16.

43. R.A. Smith & C.Baglioni (1987) The active form of tumor necrosis factor is a trimer. *J Biol Chem* 262, 6951-4.

44. B.B. Aggarwal (1992) Tumor Necrosis Factor. In: Human cytokines. Eds: Aggarwal B.B., Gutterman J.U., Blackwell Scientific Publications, Boston, MA.

45. B. Beutler & A. Cerami (1988) The common mediator of shock, cachexia, and tumor necrosis. *Adv Immunol* 42, 213-31.

46. N.L. Paul & N.H. Ruddle (1988) Lymphotoxin. *Ann Rev Immunol* 6, 407-38.

47. T. Miethke, H. Gaus, C. Wahl, K. Heeg & H. Wagner (1992) T-cell-dependent shock induced by a bacterial superantigen. *Chem Immunol* 55, 172-84.

48. T. Miethke, C. Wahl, K. Heeg, B. Echtenacher, P.H. Krammer & H. Wagner (1992) T cell-mediated lethal shock triggered in mice by the superantigen staphylococcal enterotoxin B: critical role of tumor necrosis factor. *J Exp Med* 175, 91-8.

49. J. Van Snick: Interleukin-6 (1990) An overview. *Annu Rev Immunol* 8, 253-78.

50. T. Hirano (1992) The biology of interleukin-6. *Chem Immunol* 51, 153-80.

51. T. Hirano, T. Taga, T. Matsuda, M. Hibi, S. Suematsu, B. Tang, M. Murakami & T. Kishimoto (1990) Interleukin 6 and its receptor in the immune response and hematopoiesis. *Int J Cell Cloning* 8, 155-66.

52. T. Hirano (1992) Interleukin-6 and its relation to inflammation and disease. *Clin Immunol Immunopathol* 62, 60-5.

53. P.L.J. Tan, S. Farmiloe, S. Yeoman & J.D. Watson (1990) Expression of the interleukin 6 gene in rheumatoid synovial fibroblasts. *J Rheumatol* 17, 1608-12.

54. C.A. Feghali, K.L. Bost, D.W. Boulware & L.S. Levy (1992) Mechanisms of pathogenesis in scleroderma. I. Overproduction of IL-6 by fibroblasts cultured from affected skin sites of patients with scleroderma. *J Rheumatol* 19, 1207-11.

55. S.R. Paul & P. Schendel (1992) The cloning and biological characterization of recombinant human interleukin 11. *Int J Cell Cloning* 10, 135-43.

56. H. Baumann & P. Schendel (1991) Interleukin-11 regulates the hepatic expression of the same plasma protein genes as interleukin-6. *J Biol chem* 266, 20424-27.

57. M.D. Miller & M.S. Krangel (1992) Biology and biochemistry of the chemokines: a family of chemotactic and inflammatory cytokines, *Crit Rev Immunol* 12, 17-46.

58. M.Y. Stoeckle & K.A. Barker (1990) Two burgeoning families of platelet factor 4-related proteins: mediators of the inflammatory response, *New Biologist* 2, 313-23.

59. R.M. Strieter, T.J. Standiford, G.B. Huffnagle, L.M. Colletti, N.W. Lukacs & S.L. Kunke (1996) The Good, the Bad, and the Ugly. The role of chemokines in models of human disease. *J Immunol* 156, 3583-86.

60. M. Baggiolini & I. Clark-Lewis (1992) Interleukin-8, a chemotactic and inflammatory cytokine. *FEBS Lett* 307, 97-101.

61. J. Van Damme (1994) Interleukin-8 and related chemotactic cytokines. In: The Cytokine Handbook. Ed: Thomson A., Academic Press, San Diego, CA

62. A.R. Huber, S.L. Kunkel, R.F. Todd 3d & S.J. Weiss (1991) Regulation of transendothelial neutrophil migration by endogenous interleukin-8. *Science* 254, 99-102.

63. M. Seitz, B. Dewald, M. Ceska, N. Gerber & M. Baggiolini (1992) Interleukin-8 in inflammatory rheumatic diseases: synovial fluid levels, relation to rheumatoid factors, production by mononuclear cells, and effects of gold sodium thiomalate and methotrexate. *Rheumatol Int* 12, 159-64.

64. Y.R. Mahida, M. Ceska, F. Effenberger, L. Kurlak, I. Lindley & C.J. Hawkey (1992) Enhanced synthesis of neutrophil-activating peptide-1/ interleukin-8 in active ulcerative colitis. *Clin Sci* 82, 273-5.

65. S.L. Kunkel, N. Lukacs, T. Kasama & R.M. Strieter (1996) The role of chemokines in inflammatory joint disease. *J Leukoc Biol* 58, 6-12.

66. E.A. Garcia-Zepeda, M.E. Rothenberg, R.T. Ownbey, J. Celestin, P. Leder & A.D. Luster (1996) Human eotaxin is a specific chemoattractant for eosinophil cells and provides a new mechanism to explain tissue eosinophilia. *Nature Med* 2, 449-56.

67. S. Laberge, W.W. Cruikshank, D.J. Beer & D.M. Center (1996) Secretion of IL-16 (Lymphocyte chemoattractant factor) from serotonin-stimulated CD8+ T cells in vitro. *J Immunol* 156, 310-15.

68. W.W. Cruikshank, D.M. Center, N. Nisar, M. Wu, B. Natke, A.C. Theodore & H. Kornfeld (1994) Molecular and functional analysis of a lymphocyte chemoattractant factor. Association of biologic function with CD4 expression. *Proc Natl Acad Sci USA* 91, 5109-13.

69. G.S. Kelner, J. Kennedy, K.B. Bacon, S. Kleyensteuber, D.A. Largaespada, N.A. Jenkins, N.G. Copeland, J.F. Bazan, K.W. Moore, T.J. Schall & A. Zlotnik (1994) Lymphotactin: a cytokine that represents a new class of chemokine. *Science* 266, 1395-9.

70. W.W. Cruikshank, A. Long, R.E. Tarpy, H. Kornfeld, M.P. Carroll, L. Teran, S.T. Holgate & D.M. Center (1995) Early identification of interleukin-16 (lymphocyte chemoattractant factor) and macrophage inflammatory protein 1 alpha (MIP-1a) in bronchoalveolar lavage fluid of antigen-challenged asthmatics. *Am J Resp Cell Mol Biol* 13, 738-47.

71. Z. Yao, S.L. Painter, W.C. Fanslow, D. Ulrich, B.M. Macduff, M.K. Spriggs & R.J. Armitage (1995) Human IL-17: a novel cytokine derived from T cells. *J Immunol* 155, 5483-6

72. D. Metcalf (1990) The colony stimulating factors. Discovery, development, and clinical applications. *Cancer* 65, 2185-95.

73. S. Nagata (1994) Granulocyte colony stimulating factor and its receptor. In: The Cytokine Handbook. Ed: Thomson A., Academic Press, San Diego, CA

74. J.P. Arm & T.H. Lee (1992) The pathobiology of bronchial asthma. *Adv Immunol* 51, 323-82.

75. K. Koike, M. Ogawa, J.N. Ihle, T. Miyake, T. Shimizu, A. Miyajima, T. Yokota & K-I. Arai (1987) Recombinant murine granulocyte-macrophage (GM) colony-stimulating factor supports formation of GM and multipotential blast cell colonies in culture: comparison with the effects of interleukin-3. *J Cell Physiol* 131, 458-64

76. J.W. Schrader (1994) Interleukin-3. In: The Cytokine Handbook. Ed: Thomson A., Academic Press, San Diego, CA

77. K.-I. Arai, F. Lee, A. Miyajima, S. Miyatake, N. Arai & T. Yokota (1991) Cytokines: coordinators of immune and inflammatory responses. *Annu Rev Biochem* 59, 783-836.

78. P.S.Crosier & S.C. Clark (1992) Basic biology of the hematopoietic growth factors. *Semin Oncol* 19, 349- 61.

79. M.P. Beckmann, D. Cosman, W. Fanslow, C.R. Maliszewski & S.D. Lyman (1992) The interleukin-4 receptor: structure, function, and signal transduction. *Chem Immunol* 51, 107-34.

80. T. Yokota, N. Arai, J. De Vries, H. Spits, J. Banchereau, A. Zlotnik, D. Rennick, M. Howard, Y. Takebe, S. Miyatake, F. Lee & K-I. Arai (1988) Molecular biology of interleukin 4 and interleukin 5 genes and biology of their products that stimulate B cells, T cells, and hemopoietic cells. *Immunol Rev* 102, 137- 87.

81. R. Kuhn, K. Rajewsky & W. Muller (1991) Generation and analysis of interleukin-4 deficient mice. *Science* 254, 707-10.

82. C. Fertin, J.F. Nicolas, P. Gillery, B. Kalis, J. Banchereau & F.X. Maquart (1991) Interleukin-4 stimulates collagen synthesis by normal and scleroderma fibroblasts in dermal equivalents. *Cell Mol Biol* 37, 823-9.

83. C.A. Feghali, K.L. Bost, D.W. Boulware & L.S. Levy (1992) Human recombinant interleukin-4 induces proliferation and interleukin-6 production by cultured human skin fibroblasts. *Clin Immunol Immunopathol* 63, 182-7

84. P. Miossec (1993) Interleukin 4. A potential anti-inflammatory agent. *Rev Rheum* 60, 119-24

85. R.G. Goodwin, S. Lupton, A. Schmierer, K.J. Hjerrild, R. Jerzy, W. Clevenger, S. Gillis, D. Cosman & A.E. Namen (1989)Human interleukin-7: molecular cloning and growth factor activity on human and murine B-lineage cells. *Proc Natl Acad Sci USA* 86, 302-6.

86. J. Van Snick, A. Goethals, J.C. Renauld, E. Van Roost, C. Uyttenhove, M.R. Rubira, R.L. Moritz & R.J. Simpson (1989) Cloning and characterization of a cDNA for a new mouse T cell growth factor (P40). *J Exp Med* 169, 363-8.

87. Y.C. Yang, S. Ricciardi, A. Ciarletta, J. Calvetti, K. Kelleher & S.C. Clark (1989). Expression cloning of cDNA encoding a novel human hematopoietic growth factor: human homologue of murine T-cell growth factor P40. *Blood* 74, 1880-4.

88. K. Kelleher, K. Bean, S.C. Clark, W.Y. Leung, T.L. Yang-Feng, J.W. Chen, P.F. Lin, W. Luo & Y.C. Yang YC (1991) Human interleukin-9: genomic sequence, chromosomal location, and sequences essential for its expression in human T-cell leukemia virus (HTLV)-I-transformed human T cells. *Blood* 77, 1436-41.

89. F.A. Houssiau, J.C. Renauld, W.E. Fibbe & J. Van Snick (1992) IL-2 dependence of IL-9 expression in human T lymphocytes. *J Immunol* 148, 3147-51.

90. M.C. Cohen & S. Cohen (1996) Cytokine Function. A study in biologic diversity. *Am J Clin Pathol* 105, 589-98.

91. W.F. Chen & A. Zlotnik (1991) IL-10: a novel cytotoxic T cell differentiation factor. *J Immunol* 147, 528-34.

92. R. de Waal Malefyt, H. Yssel, M.G. Roncarolo, H. Spits & J.E. de Vries (1992) Interleukin-10. *Curr Opin Immunol* 4, 314-20.

93. T.R. Mosmann & K.W. Moore (1991) The role of IL-10 in crossregulation of TH1 and TH2 responses. *Immunol Today* 12, A49-53.

94. K.W. Moore, P. Vieira, D.F. Fiorentino, M.L. Troustine, T.A. Khan & T.R. Mosmann (1990) Homology of cytokine synthesis inhibitory factor (IL10) to the Epstein-Barr virus gene BCRF1. *Science* 248, 1230-4.

95. T.R. Mosmann (1994) Interleukin-10. In: The Cytokine Handbook. Ed: Thomson A., Academic Press, San Diego, CA.

96. K.D. Brown, S.M. Zurawski, T.R. Mosmann & G. Zurawski (1989) A family of small inducible proteins secreted by leukocytes are members of a new superfamily that includes leukocyte and fibroblastderived inflammatory agents, growth factors, and indicators of various activation processes. *J Immunol* 142, 679-87.

97. Minty, P. Chalon, J.M. Derocq, X. Dumont, J.C. Guillemot, M. Kaghad, C. Labit, P. Leplatois, P. Liauzun, B. Miloux, C. Minty, P. Casellas, G. Loison, J. Lupker, D. Shire, P. Ferrara & D. Caput (1993) Interleukin-13 is a new human lymphokine regulating inflammatory and immune responses. *Nature* 362, 248-50.

98. J. Punnonen, G. Aversa, B.G. Cocks, A.N. McKenzie, S. Menon, G. Zurawski, R. de Waal Malefyt & J.E. de Vries JE (1993) Interleukin 13 induces interleukin 4-independent IgG4 and IgE synthesis and CD23 expression by human B cells. *Proc Natl Acad Sci USA* 90, 3730-4.

99. R. Ford, A. Tamayo, B. Martin, K. Niu, K. Claypool, F. Cabanillas & J. Ambrus Jr (1995) Identification of B-cell growth factors (interleukin-14; high molecular weight-B-cell growth factors) in effusion fluids from patients with aggressive B-cell lymphomas. *Blood* 86, 283-93.

100. M.B. Sporn, A.B. Roberts, L.M. Wakefield & R.K. Assoian RK (1986) Transforming growth factor: biological function and chemical structure. *Science* 233, 532-4.

101. W.O. Cooper, R.A. Fava, C.A. Gates, M.A. Cremer & A.S. Townes (1992) Acceleration of onset of collagen-induced arthritis by

intra-articular injection of tumour necrosis factor or transforming growth factor-beta. *Clin Exp Immunol* 89, 244-50.

102. H.G. Herrod (1989) Interleukins in immunologic and allergic diseases. *Ann Allergy* 63, 269-72

103. M.K. Gately, A.G. Wolitzky, P.M. Quinn & R. Chizzonite (1992) Regulation of human cytolytic lymphocyte responses by interleukin-12. *Cell Immunol* 143, 127- 42.

104. M. Kiniwa, M. Gately, U. Gubler, R. Chizzonite, C. Fargeas & G. Delespesse (1992) Recombinant interleukin-12 suppresses the synthesis of immunoglobulin E by interleukin-4 stimulated human lymphocytes. *J Clin Invest* 90, 262-6.

105. P. Scott (1993) IL-12: initiation cytokine for cellmediated immunity. *Science* 260, 496-7.

106. J.G. Giri, D.M. Anderson, S. Kumaki, L.S. Park, K.H. Grabstein & D. Cosman (1995) IL-15, a novel T cell growth factor that shares activities and receptor components with IL-2. *J Leukoc Biol* 57, 763-6.

107. T.M. Doherty, R.A. Seder & A. Sher (1996) Induction and regulation of IL-15 expression in murine macrophages. *J Immunol* 156, 735-41.

108. I.B. McInnes, J. Al-Mughales, M. Field, B.P. Leung, F.P. Huang, R. Dixon, R.D. Sturrock, P.C. wilkinson & F.Y. Liew (1996) The role of interleukin-15 in T-cell migration and activation in rheumatoid arthritis. *Nature Med* 2, 175-82.

109. E.F. Wheelock (1965) Interferon-like virus-inhibitor induced in human leukocytes by phytohemagglutinin. *Science* 149, 310-11.

110. E. De Maeyer & J. De Maeyer-Guignard (1994) Interferons. In: The Cytokine Handbook. Ed: Thomson A., Academic Press, San Diego, CA.

111. H. Heremans & A. Billiau (1989) The potential role of interferons and interferon antagonists in inflammatory disease. *Drugs* 38, 957-72.

112. 76. C.O. Jacob, P.H. van der Meide & H.O. McDevitt (1987) In vivo treatment of (NZB x NZW)F1 lupus-like nephritis with monoclonal antibody to interferon. *J Exp Med* 166, 798-803.

113. I.L. Campbell, L. Oxbrow, M. Koulmanda & L.C. Harrison (1988) IFN-?induces islet cell MHC antigens and enhances autoimmune, streptozotocin-induced diabetes in the mouse. *J Immunol* 140, 1111-6.

114. N. Sarvetnick, D. Liggitt, S.L. Pitts, S.E. Hansen & T.A. Stewart (1988) Insulin-dependent diabetes mellitus induced in transgenic mice by ectopic expression of class II MHC and interferon-gamma. *Cell* 52, 773-82.

115. N.J. Mauritz, R. Holdmdahl, R. Jonsson, P.H. van der Meide, A. Scheynius & L. Klareskog (1988) Treatment with gamma-interferon triggers the onset of collagen arthritis in mice. *Arthritis Rheum* 31, 1297-1304.

116. G.E. Grau, H. Heremans, P.F. Piguet, P. Pointaire, P.H. Lambert, A. Billiau & P. Vassalli (1989) Monoclonal antibody against interferon ?can prevent experimental cerebral malaria and its associated overproduction of tumor necrosis factor. *Proc Natl Acad Sci USA* 86, 55724.

117. D.K. Dalton, S. Pitts-Meek, S. Keshav, I.S. Figari, A. Bradley & T.A. Stewart (1993) Multiple defects of immune cell function in mice with disrupted interferon-gamma genes. *Science* 259, 1739-42.

118. H. Okamura, H. Tsutsui, T. Komatsu, M. Yutsudo, A. Hakura, T. Tanimoto, K. Torigoe, T. Okura, Y. Nukada, K. Hattori, K. Akita, M. Namba, F. Tanabe, K. Konishi, S. Fukuda, & M. Kurimoto (1995) Cloning of a new cytokine that induces IFN- production by T cells. *Science* 378, 88-91.

119. S. Ushio, M. Namba, T. Okura, K. Hattori, Y. Nukada, K. Akita, F. Tanabe, K. Konishi, M. Micallef, M. Fuji, K. Torigoe, T. Tanimoto, S. Fukuda, M. Ikeda, H. Okamura, & M. Kurimoto (1996) Cloning of the cDNA for human IFN-inducing factor, expression in *Escherichia coli*, and studies on the biologic activities of the protein. *J Immunol* 156, 4274-9.

120. T. Kishimoto, S. Akira & T. Taga (1992) Interleukin-6 and its receptor: a paradigm for cytokines. *Science* 258, 593-7.

121. W.C. Greene (1986) The human interleukin-2 receptor. *Annu Rev Immunol* 4, 69-95.

122. K.A. Smith (1999) The two-chain structure of highaffinity IL-2 receptors. *Immunol Today* 8, 11-13.

123. M.N. Manoussakis, G.K. Papadopoulos, A.A. Drosos & H.M. Moutsopoulos (1989) Soluble interleukin 2 receptor molecules in the serum of patients with autoimmune diseases. *Clin Immunol Immunopathol* 50, 321-32.

124. T. Taga, M. Hibi, M. Murakami, M. Saito, H. Yawata, M. Narazaki, Y. Hirata, T. Sugita, K. Yasukawa, T. Hirano & T. Kishimoto (1992) Interleukin-6 receptor and signals. *Chem Immunol* 51, 181-204.

125. J.F. Bazan (1990) Structural design and molecular evolution of a cytokine receptor superfamily. *Proc Natl Acad Sci USA* 87, 6934-8.

126. Oehm, I. Behrmann, W. Falk, M. Pawlita, G. Maier, C. Klas, M. Li-Weber, S. Richards, J. Dhein, B.C. Trauth, H. Ponstingl & P.H. Krammer (1992) Purification and molecular cloning of the APO-1 cell surface antigen, a member of the tumor necrosis factor/nerve growth factor receptor superfamily: sequence identity with the Fas antigen. *J Biol Chem* 267, 10709-15.

127. J. Banchereau, F. Bazan, D. Blanchard, F. Briere, J.P. Galizzi, C. van Kooten, Y.J. Liu, F. Rousset, & S. Saeland (1994) The CD40 antigen and its ligand. *Annu Rev Immunol* 12, 881-922.

128. L.A. Tartaglia & D.V. Goeddel (1992) Two TNF receptors. *Immunol Today* 13, 151-3.

129. K. Wiegmann, S. Schutze, E. Kampen, A. Himmler, T. Machleidt & M. Kronke (1992) Human 55-kDa receptor for tumor necrosis factor coupled to signal transduction cascades. *J Biol Chem* 267, 17997-8001.

130. T.N.C. Wells, C.A. Power, M. Lusti-Narasimhan, A.J. Hoogewerf, R.M. Cooke, C. Chung, M.C. Peitsch & A.E.I. Proudfoot (1996) Selectivity and antagonism of chemokine receptors. *J Leukoc Biol* 59, 53-60.

131. C.J. Raport, V.L. Schweickart, D. Chantry, R.L. Eddy Jr., T.B. Shows, R. Godiska & P.W. Gray (1996) New members of the chemokine receptor gene family. *J Leuko. Biol* 59, 18-23.

132. P. Bates (1996) Chemokine receptors and HIV-1: an attractive pair? *Cell* 86, 1-3.

133. M. Dean, M. Carrington, C. Winkler, G.A. Huttley, M.W. Smith, R. Allidmets, J.I. Goedert, S.P. Buchbinder, E. Vittinghoff, E. Gomperts, S. Donfield, D. Vlahov, R. Kaslow, A. Saah, C. Rinaldo & R. Detels (1996) Genetic restriction of HIV-1 infection and progression to AIDS by a deletion allele of the *CKR5* structural gene. *Science* 273, 1856-62.

Index